MUD
SALT

+

MEDICINE

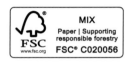

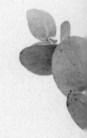

Published in 2023 by OH! Life
An imprint of Welbeck Non-Fiction Limited,
part of Welbeck Publishing Group.
Offices in London, 20 Mortimer Street, London W1T 3JW,
and Sydney, 205 Commonwealth Street, Surry Hills 2010
www.welbeckpublishing.com

A CIP catalogue record for this book is available from
the British Library.

ISBN 978-1-83861-089-0

Associate Publisher: Lisa Dyer
Copyeditor: Katie Hewett
Designer: Georgie Hewitt
Production Controller: Felicity Awdry

Printed and bound in China

10 9 8 7 6 5 4 3 2 1

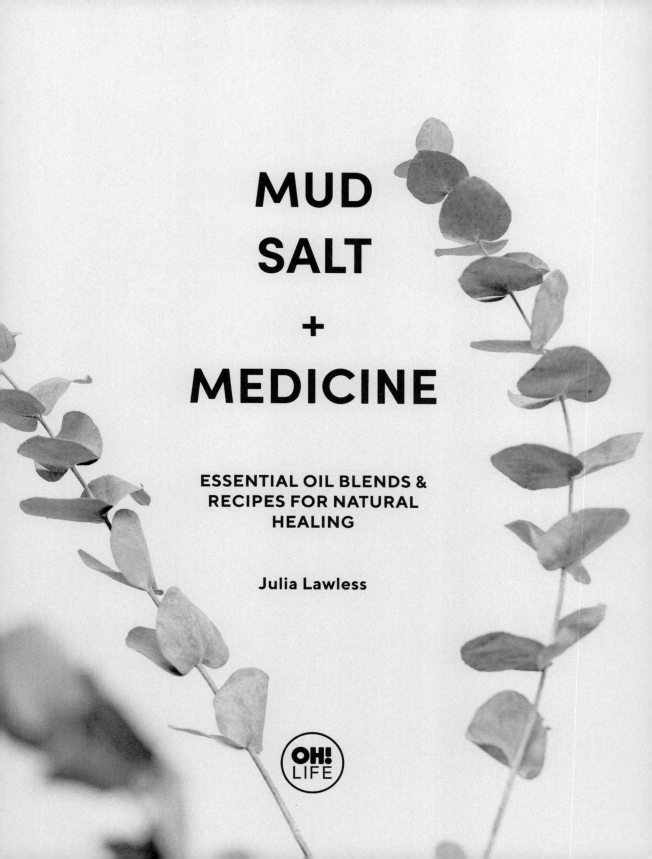

MUD
SALT
+
MEDICINE

ESSENTIAL OIL BLENDS & RECIPES FOR NATURAL HEALING

Julia Lawless

OH!
LIFE

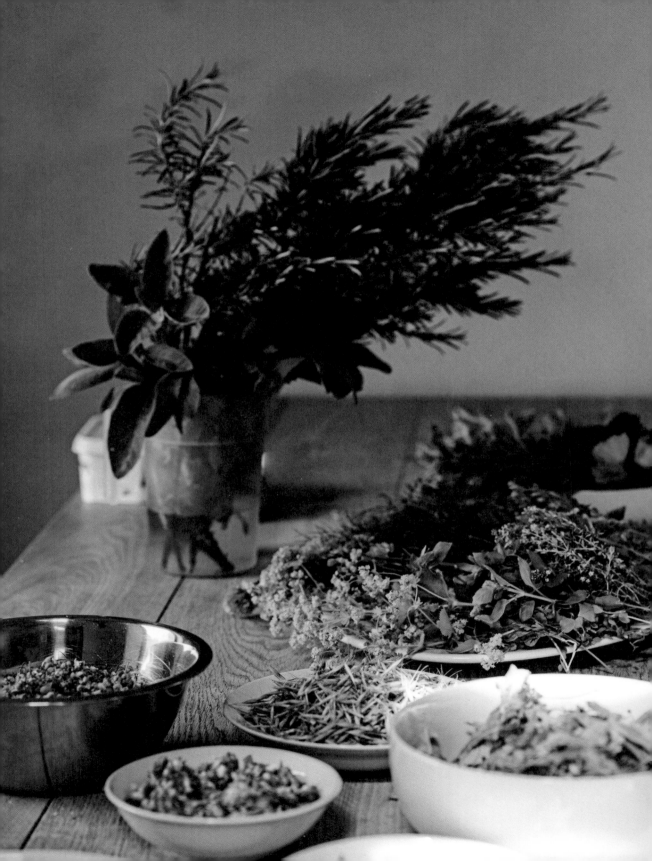

CONTENTS

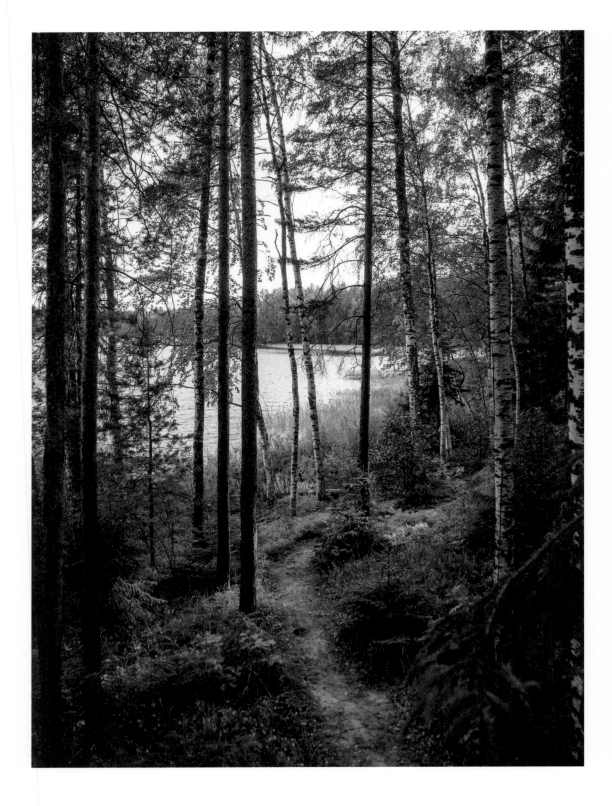

PREFACE

I inherited the knowledge of using plants, herbs and oils from the maternal side of my family. A strong connection with nature and wilderness still exists in Finland because it is a place where the landscape is dominated by vast forests, sea inlets and numerous lakes. My mother Kerttu Ajanko, a Finnish biochemist, was involved in the research of essential oils and the healing potential of natural aromatics in Helsinki long before the term 'aromatherapy' became fashionable. Luckily, I still have many of my mother's own recipes for creating aromatic products at home. Her notebooks include how to make creams and balms, as well as many other innovative aromatic products, such as blended flower waters and lotions. As a research chemist, she was familiar with using hands-on techniques, which included producing her own essential oils using a simple distillation method, and I can still remember her experimenting with all sorts of potions on our kitchen table when I was a child.

Mud, Salt + Medicine is based on the fundamental principle of using only pure, botanical ingredients to create effective and environmentally friendly products. In this book I share some of my personal experience and expertise in creating unique aromatic products, for over 30 years, for our family business Aqua Oleum. This book can be used both as an inspirational source for discovering new recipes and blending ideas or as a reference manual covering a wide range of aromatic oils and natural materials. Here, I focus on the formulation process itself and describe the various step-by-step processes by which essential oils can be used in combination with other plant materials, such as botanical carrier oils, herbal infusions, flower waters, waxes, clays and salts, to make a range of aromatic preparations and health-enhancing treatments and remedies.

You will also learn how to create an aromatic sanctuary within your own home – a place to relax, renew and cleanse both your body and your mind. Simply relaxing in a warm aromatic bath, while utilizing certain salts, clays, oils and herbs for their specific healing properties, is a therapy in itself. Knowing that this is an ancient ritual, which has been practised for thousands of years by all cultures alike using 100 per cent natural ingredients, makes it part of a universal human experience. I hope the ideas and recipes in this book will therefore help inspire you to make something amazing with your own hands – often at a fraction of the cost of a ready-made item – while at the same time enhancing personal creativity, health and wellbeing.

Julia Lawless

INTRODUCTION
HEALING THROUGH NATURE

'Health is the expression of a harmonious balance between the various components of human nature, the environment and ways of life: nature is the physician of disease.' **HIPPOCRATES**

Botanical plants and aromatic herbs, together with other natural materials such as mud, salt, oil and water, constitute the basis for our original medicines. At one time, the knowledge of how to utilize these naturally occurring substances for sustenance and healing was passed down through the generations as a valuable living experience: plants with medicinal properties were used by early prehistoric humans as an intrinsic part of their hunter-gatherer lifestyle. Ancient records and folklore also bear witness to a whole range of plants being used for ritual purposes, cosmetics and as remedies within diverse communities across the globe. For thousands of years, the Aboriginal Australians have used the twigs of tea tree (*Melaleuca alternifolia*) for healing wounds and treating infection; in the New World, the Native Americans traditionally used the smoke from bundles of 'sacred sage' (*Salvia apiana*) in their sweat lodges to purify the body and spirit — the leaves were also made into a herbal tea to combat coughs and respiratory infections; while in Egypt, the aromatic gum resins

of frankincense (*Boswellia carteri*) and myrrh (*Commiphora myrrha*) were burned as precious incense or combined with waxes and oils for embalming their kings and healing their warriors. Still today, many of our modern drugs are derived directly from plants: for example, morphine is made from the dried latex found within the seed pods of the opium poppy (*Papaver somniferum*), having been used as a medicine since Neolithic times; and quinine from the bark of the Peruvian tree (*Cinchona officinalis*) was traditionally used by South American tribes for reducing fever.

The naturopathic movement, which was first practised around 400 BCE by the Hippocratic School of Medicine, was based on an inherent respect for nature. The Greek philosopher Hippocrates believed that it was important to view the whole person when identifying the cause of a particular disease, and in using the laws of nature to induce a cure. Naturopathy, or Nature Cure, is underpinned by a fundamental belief in the healing powers of nature.

Hippocrates maintained that we are an intrinsic part of nature, and that good health is achieved by living in accordance with this understanding. Harmony is fostered though proper nutrition, herbal treatments, aromatic massage, bathing, rest, sunshine and fasting. Medicine, science and religion were intimately interconnected – and humankind was seen as a whole: as a physical, mental, emotional and spiritual being. Early naturopaths believed that if we could simply restore our vital life-force, the body would naturally heal itself. Hippocrates therefore recommended a daily aromatic bath followed by a massage using aromatic oils as the way to both enhance and restore optimum health. However, the primary focus was on taking preventative measures against disease in the first place, so in many ways, naturopathy looked to the raw elements themselves for their revitalizing and life-giving qualities.

Based on these same principles, people from all parts of the world have utilized the therapeutic benefits of thermal springs and baths as part of an age-old tradition. Gradually, certain individuals realized that bathing in these mineral-rich hot springs was not only relaxing, but also offered a range of other health benefits. Hot water can hold more dissolved solids than cold water, including mud, clay and salt, as well as containing a range of minerals that have healing benefits. While bathing in a hot spring, the body naturally absorbs trace amounts of the minerals found in the water via the pores of the skin, such as sulphur,

calcium, magnesium and lithium. These trace minerals help provide healing effects to different organs and systems in the body, as well as acting as a natural remedy for a range of skin conditions. Over time, and based on the natural terrain of each location, different types of spa tradition developed right across the globe, each with their own rituals and therapeutic methods of treatment. Many of these are very ancient and have their origins in early systems of belief, where humanity and the natural world were perceived as being inter-related and interdependent.

The Indian ayurvedic system, from the Sanskrit meaning 'knowledge for long life', is part of an ancient Hindu tradition based on healing principles that seek to improve health and wellbeing by creating a balance between mind, body and spirit through an assessment of overall lifestyle. Treatments are based on herbal preparations, diet, fasting, purification, meditation and yoga – all entirely natural techniques. It is one of the oldest forms of healthcare in the world and is all-encompassing in its approach to wellness. Taking time for personal reflection and self-understanding is also encouraged by leaving the outside world behind and entering a serene oasis or place of retreat for a while, so it is possible to focus on restoring physical and emotional equilibrium from within. Simply spending time outdoors in nature – walking, gardening, bird watching or just doing whatever hobby or sport you enjoy – can also provide relief from the everyday pressures of work and recharge your batteries. The healing power and potential of simply being in a natural environment has been scientifically verified in recent years. However, since it is not always possible to get away or spend time in nature, we can always create a healing sanctuary within our own homes to promote a sense of renewal and regeneration using natural materials.

Creating a home sanctuary does not need to be expensive or complicated – it is more about making a mental decision to set time aside for oneself. And, of course, good health and longevity is not just about reducing wrinkles and looking good from the outside; it is also about prolonging vitality and promoting an optimum sense of wellbeing psychologically. This means having a positive mental attitude and developing a feeling of emotional equilibrium in our lives as well as enjoying a sense of basic contentment. Developing meditation, mindfulness and breathing practices have been shown to help with mental health issues and to support our inner quality of life by helping us to relax and deal with problems such as stress, anxiety and depression. If we can appreciate what we have and focus on the present moment, this can be a powerful antidote to dwelling on the past or worrying about the future. When we combine these types of meditative approach with those focused on the body, such as improving the quality of our nutrition and ensuring we get enough exercise,

then we can be sure we are taking a holistic view of our own health.

In addition, skincare and rejuvenating treatments, such as massage, body scrubs and exfoliation treatments, can also enhance this process, especially when personalized to your individual condition. Many of the naturopathic traditions therefore developed specific healing treatments to increase circulation, remove toxins, promote a youthful skin and generally optimize wellbeing and longevity. For example, the ayurvedic healing system traditionally uses a silk-mitt exfoliation technique to soften the skin; the Roman *thermae* custom encourages dry skin brushing to stimulate the circulation and remove fatty deposits; while the sauna tradition employs a *vihta*, a bundle of supple birch twigs, to gently beat the surface of the skin to encourage sweating, open the pores and remove toxins.

I grew up accustomed to using a traditional outdoor sauna, which is heated with a wood-burning stove. This is generally built next to the sea or beside a lake since these are plentiful in Finland. The sauna shares many of the same ritual elements as other age-old traditional customs, such as the Native American sweat lodge. What can be more primal than breaking the ice and swimming in the freezing water of a Finnish inlet or rolling in the snow at midwinter! The Finnish sauna is fundamentally a dry heat experience, which can be seen as a variant of the steam bath or wet heat alternative now popularized as

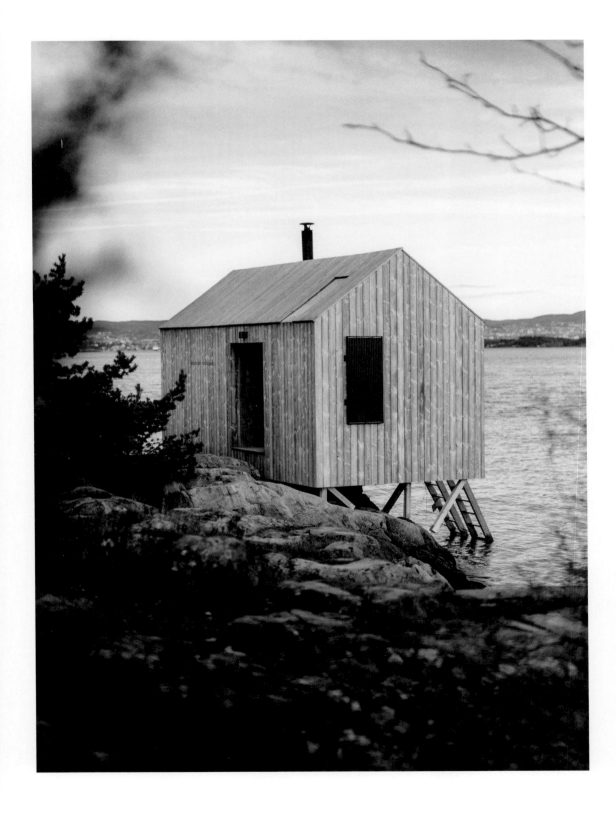

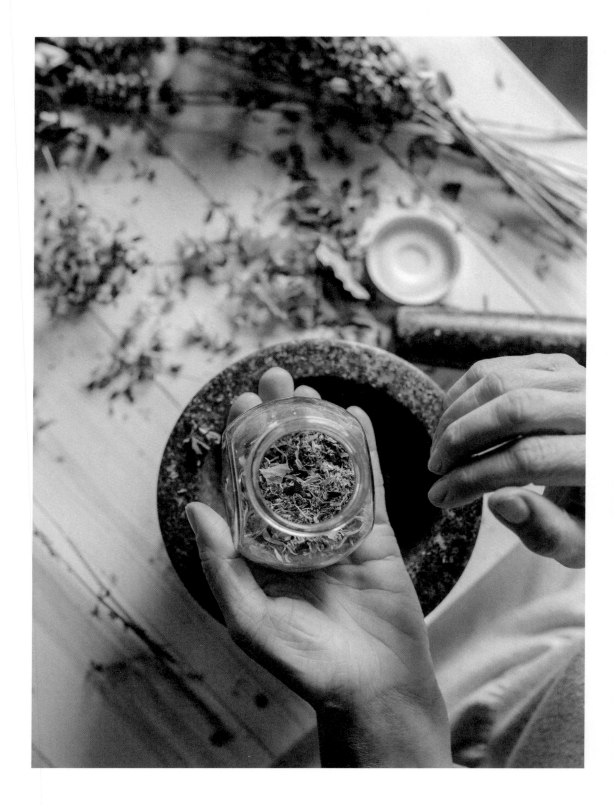

the Turkish hammam. The hammam experience also commonly utilizes deep tissue massage and a deep cleanse using an aromatic black soap with essential oils. The oils are also infused into the air, as they are in the sauna, so as the steam is absorbed through the pores, the aromatic oils help to purify and relax us.

Today with the holistic movement gaining popularity, many people are turning for guidance to the philosophies and principles illustrated by these various naturalistic healing traditions. Aromatherapy, which uses aromatic oils in massage, skincare, steam inhalation and for general physical and emotional wellbeing, specifically embodies many of the techniques of these early therapeutic models, which includes the use of mud, salt and water treatments. It is also important to point out that by using natural materials and techniques that have been tried and tested for hundreds of years – often for thousands of years – this does not mean that these methods are any less potent or active than many of the scientifically engineered products which are available today. As Imelda Burke says in her book *The Nature of Beauty*:

'There is NO LESS science in a natural product than a synthetic one. In fact, much of the science that mainstream brands will talk about, is from the latest plant discovery they have made and are using as their key active ingredient: here is the thing – nature IS science.'

Certainly, it has become apparent that the commercial exploitation of the Earth's resources that has depleted the planet's wildlife and has polluted our environment across land, sea and air has largely arisen due to a profound disrespect for the natural world. The use of petrochemical products, such as mineral oil found as a principal ingredient in many mainstream cosmetics, is amplifying the effects of climate change through the continued burning of fossil fuels. The use of synthetic microbeads in many toiletries, such as soaps and exfoliants, which then find their way into the water systems, are poisoning our oceans and the marine life within them (they were banned in the UK in 2021). The superfluous packaging and by-products involved in the production of many beauty and perfumery items also contributes to the build-up of non-biodegradable waste, which ends up in toxic landfills. In contrast, by creating homemade products using natural and recyclable materials, we can help to turn the tide back on our currently unsustainable and unecological way of living. Faced with the implications of climate change, our fast-fix way of life, which does not take heed of the consequences of our present-day actions further down the line, is now untenable. Today, we are urgently faced with finding new ways of approaching our everyday habits and rituals through learning to live in harmony with nature, both as individuals and as part of our global community.

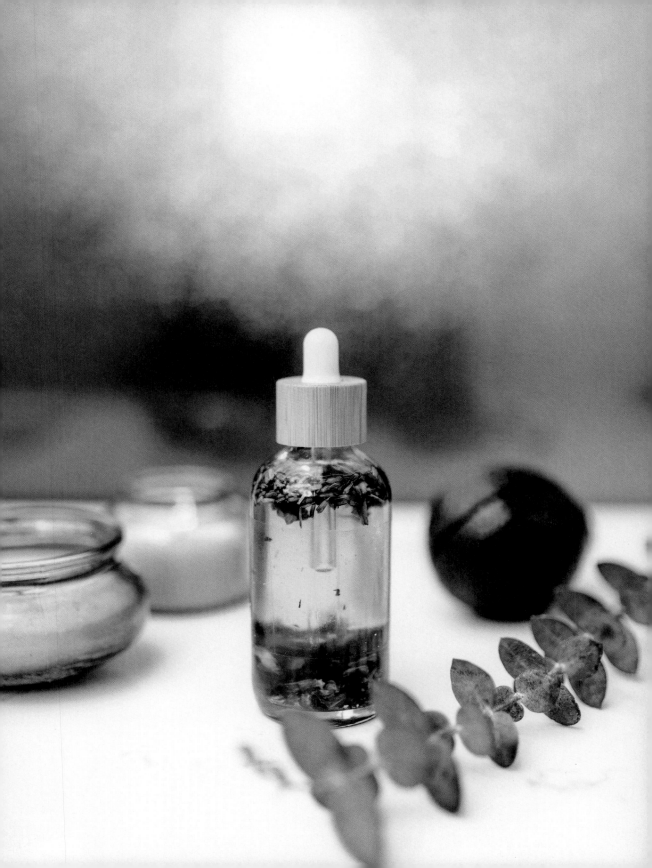

AROMATIC

TREATMENTS, BLENDS

+ RECIPES

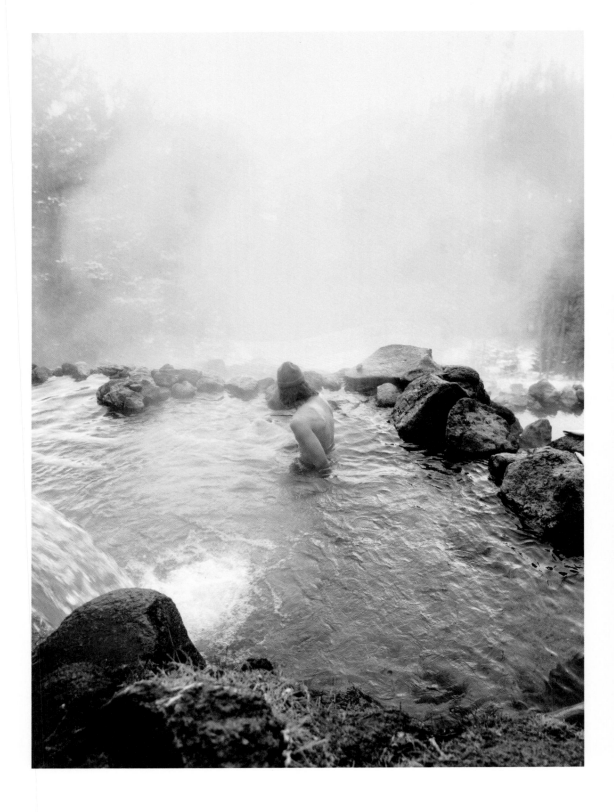

'I am sure there are things that can't be cured by a good bath, but I can't think of one...'

SYLVIA PLATH, *THE BELL JAR*

1 + BATHING

Thermal Bathing + the Spa Tradition

Bathing in thermal water is one of the earliest therapeutic practices. The origin of the word 'spa' is from the Latin phrase *salus per aquaem*, meaning simply 'health through water'. The pleasurable and healing experience of soaking in the warm water of a natural hot spring constitutes the original basis for the development of the spa tradition. A hot spring is essentially formed as a by-product of being located near a high concentration of volcanic or geothermal energy where super-heated water erupts from the Earth's crust. As the water forces its way upwards, it absorbs the rich mineral deposits found in the surrounding rock and earth, which are consequently found in large quantities dissolved in the hot spring's water.

Hot springs can be found all over the world and each culture has developed their own unique ways of enjoying their benefits where the mineral content of each spring offers healing qualities specific to that one place. According to the principles of Chinese medicine, a hot spring passes on the *qi* or the life-force energy of all five elements: earth, water, wood, fire and metal, in the form of the various minerals found in the water of that region. Natural hot springs are often situated in very beautiful and remote locations, such as those found in the icy, lunar landscapes of Iceland or in the Rocky Mountains of Colorado. I have visited several hot springs in Colorado where it is customary to walk several miles through the mountain wilderness before reaching a secluded thermal pool or spring. This type of naturalistic bathing experience not only gives the body and mind a chance to repair itself via the healing waters but also enhances our sense of wellbeing through our immersion and connection with the natural environment.

The native American tribes – the Cheyenne, Ute and Arapaho – who were the first to discover the healing advantages of the mineral hot springs in their territorial lands, named these thermal areas the 'places of magic waters' due to their powerful healing benefits. In Thailand, the local hot springs were considered to have a mystical, pure significance. The sacred water from the hot springs at Ranong, for example, were traditionally used for important religious and royal ceremonies. The association of bathing with holy rites and purification also has very ancient roots. Long before the Spanish colonization of South America, the Mayans were performing sacred healing rituals inside a temazcal, an igloo-like stone structure designed to facilitate spiritual cleansing and to rid the body of toxins, much like the Native American sweat lodge. During the sweat, the Mayan shaman would pour herb-infused water over a pile of searing hot volcanic rocks, so the dome filled with fragrant steam. The entrance was then sealed with a thick blanket darkening the interior and keeping the heat in, all the while accompanied by shamanic chanting.

In early civilizations, people around the world believed that ritual bathing in the thermal water from a pool or hot spring, or via herb-infused aromatic steam, resulted in both physical and spiritual purification. Such rites existed in the early Native American, Asian, Mayan, Babylonian, Greek and Roman cultures – all these traditions reflected the ancient belief in the sacred healing and cleansing powers of water. Complex bathing rituals were also practiced in ancient Egypt and in the pre-historic cities of the Indus Valley and Aegean settlements. Alongside their natural hot springs and pools, the Aegean people even utilized bathtubs, wash basins and foot baths for their personal cleanliness – prototypes for our modern bathrooms.

Over time, each culture adopted specific bathing traditions and rituals that suited the climate and customs of their country. Japan, for example, has practiced two distinct types of bathing rituals from ancient times with their onsen and sento traditions: onsen literally means a hot spring, whereas sento refers to a public hot bath, not attached to a hot spring. These are the two relatively distinct types of therapeutic bathing traditions that developed – one based around a natural thermal spring, and the other based on either a dry heat experience, such as the Finnish sauna, on a wet heat or steam experience, such as the Middle Eastern hammam. Today, however, a spa has come to mean a whole range of elemental therapeutic experiences, which may include warm baths, showers, steam rooms, hot tubs and cold plunge pools as well as a range of other natural healing practices such as massage, body treatments and facials. The factor which they all have in common, is that they harness and utilize the simple yet powerful forces of nature and the elements as their primary tools: water, heat, salt, minerals, clay, mud, herbs and natural oils.

Historically speaking, bathing was primarily a communal and social activity rather than a solitary experience. In England, the names of many towns still reflect their origins as communal bathing places, such as the famous city of Bath, once known as Aquae Sulis, whose natural healing waters have been used for thousands of years. I have visited this magnificent bathing complex on many occasions over the years, and beneath the contemporary gloss, it is still possible to sense the sacred origins of this site with its precious thermal waters. Here, the Romans constructed a temple to the goddess Sulis Minerva: dedicated both to Sulis, the original Celtic goddess of the healing waters and Minerva, the Roman goddess of wisdom and medicine. The elaborate communal bathing complex of the Romans is dated to the middle of the first century CE, but the sacred hot spring itself was revered and worshipped from much earlier times by the local tribal people.

The Turkish bath or hammam, which was created around the same time as the Roman *thermae*, was also built on the custom of communal bathing that has evolved over thousands of years. This Middle Eastern custom is a steam heat tradition, where the key method for cleansing the body is via steam rooms of varying temperatures and the use of a unique black soap made from olive oil and eucalyptus essential oil, known as *beldi*, followed by a deep tissue massage. The Finnish sauna tradition is also a group or communal experience, having an important family and social function.

The sauna combines a dry heat experience with intermittent steam, followed by the invigorating effects of cold water. After a period spent sitting in the warmth, it is customary to plunge directly into the sea or into a lake, or if this is not possible, to take a cool shower – then this process is repeated several times. The contrast of moving from one temperature extreme to another causes a surge of blood flow that helps to circulate nutrients throughout the body. Sitting in a hot environment also causes an aerobic effect that causes the heart rate to increase and the metabolism to rise, which prompts the body to burn more calories. The high temperature of the sauna simultaneously helps to lift the spirits and boosts the metabolism in an otherwise harsh, cold environment.

Apart from the cleansing and comforting effect of the sauna's dry heat, an aromatic bundle of fresh birch twigs known as *vihta*, is traditionally used to gently beat the skin to encourage the purification process. Throwing ladles of cold water or *laulu* onto the hot stones to make bursts of steam, which encourages sweating, is also a part of the ritual. A few drops of an essential oil or a blend of oils can also be added to the *laulu* water for their therapeutic effect. Sweating flushes waste products from the muscles, leaving them rested and restored; after sweating, however, it is important always to rehydrate the body after each session to replace any water you may have lost.

My mother Kerttu was also a great advocate of dry skin brushing in the sauna washroom because the benefits are multifold. It helps exfoliation naturally by ridding the skin of dead cells and so encourages the growth of new cellular tissue; it stimulates the lymphatic system which is vital for the health of the circulation and for the elimination of toxins; and it helps to break down fatty deposits by encouraging blood flow to the surface of the skin. It also makes the texture and feel of the skin amazingly smooth and soft! Be sure to use a natural bristle brush and take about three to five minutes to work from the feet upwards towards the heart, in the direction of the natural flow of the lymphatic system.

Showers are probably the favoured bathing method for most people first thing in the morning today. But even a quick shower can become a bathing ritual by simply adding a few drops of an invigorating essential oil to the shower tray beforehand and then breathing in the aromatic vapours. Lotions, masks, scrubs, oils and body wash treatments can all be made at home using natural ingredients, many of which are best carried out prior to showering. In the ancient ayurvedic practice of *abhyanga*, a brisk body massage is followed by a warm shower. Traditionally, sesame oil was used to perform this massage, but a tablespoon of jojoba or sweet almond oil with a couple of drops of essential oils added, works equally well as a self-massage.

Immersing the whole body in a hot tub or bath has a vital healing function, simply due to the soothing and comforting effects of the warmth on our skin. Today the popularity of installing hot tubs within individual homes is on the increase, especially where the climate is cold in winter. Likewise, whirlpool baths installed with high-speed jets can provide a stimulating water-massage and help keep our body toned, in much in the same way as standing under a waterfall in a naturalistic environment. When this experience is enhanced by adding various oils, minerals, salts or clay to the water, it can mirror many of the therapeutic benefits of visiting a natural hot spring or pool. Alongside offering a wide range of health benefits, regular thermal bathing can also act as a preventative treatment. This was the basis for the great spa revival of the Victorian age in Britain where people travelled to places such as Bath or Royal Leamington Spa, to 'take the air' and enjoy the healing waters. This practice was not merely thought to bring relief to those who were already sick or who were convalescing after an illness, it was also considered to play an equally vital role as a preventative treatment.

The relaxing and healing effects of soaking in a warm bath, especially to help combat stress, depression, insomnia and all types of nervous disorders, has been well documented over the years. When mineral-rich salts or clay are added to the bath water there are further health benefits. For example, the soothing effects of warm water combined with Dead Sea salt helps to promote an overall sense of physical and mental relaxation, which reduces stress and supports our whole nervous system. Our bodies also

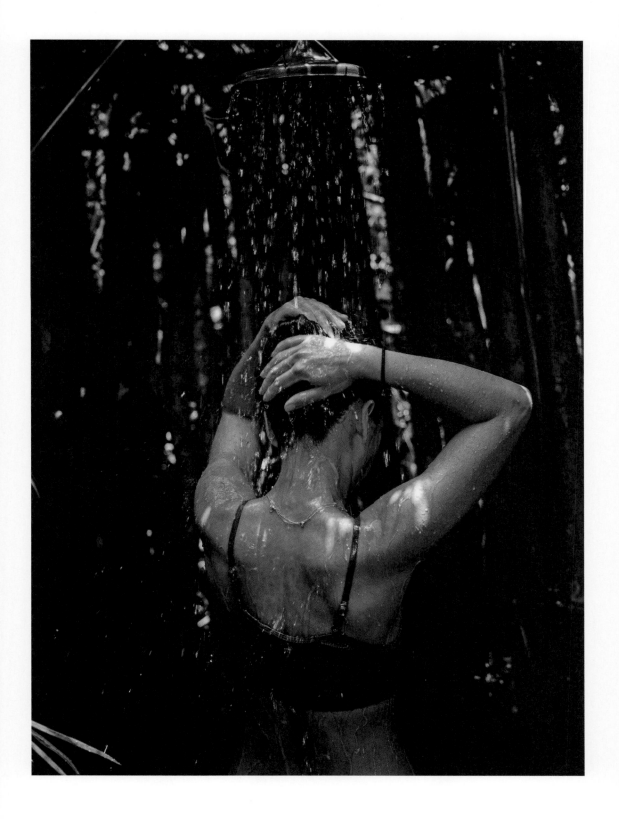

absorb minerals from the salts, which stimulates the immune system and strengthens it. These minerals enhance the production of endorphins which interact with receptors in the brain to produce a sense of wellbeing. The role of endorphins is to release positive feelings and relieve the body and mind of stress. They also help normalize glandular and hormonal function and support the immune system.

Bathing in mineral-rich waters has universally been recognized for their rejuvenating and anti-ageing properties. This is because bathing in thermal water increases the production of collagen and tightens the elastin in the cellular tissues deep within the dermis: this leaves our skin looking both firm and youthful. The main mineral responsible for this effect is silica, which is found in many of the Icelandic hot springs, such as the Blue Lagoon. Silica is also believed to restore health to ageing skin, hair and nails. Other minerals, such as calcium, lithium, magnesium and sulphur, can also help to improve the texture of the skin alongside other healing actions.

Sulphur is found in high concentrations in the natural hot springs of Tuscany in Italy, which is particularly good for healing the skin. Italy's best-known hot spring is at Saturnia in southern Tuscany where the characteristic smell of the sulphur dioxide gas escaping into the air is evident some miles away. I have been to Saturnia many times over the years, both to the wild area where the thermal water merges with the cold current of the river turning the rocks a strange whitish-yellow,

as well as to the modern spa site with its thermal swimming pool and comfortable rest rooms. The water is about 37°C (98.6°F) and instantly relaxes the body, while the minerals present in the water and clay, mainly sulphur, calcium and carbon, have been shown to help remedy a range of skin conditions. The strong presence of sulphur especially, has been shown to be effective in the treatment of eczema, dermatitis, psoriasis, rashes and even warts. Basting the body with the black, mineral-infused mud is also encouraged and leaves the skin feeling sumptuously soft. Many of these healing minerals are also found naturally in different types of clays and salts, which can be added to the bath water at home, with equally therapeutic results.

Acne is a common problem that can wreak havoc with our skin, especially in our youth. It can often be difficult to clear, yet often this unsightly condition responds well to bathing in hot water infused with healing clays, minerals and salts. Salt is naturally antiseptic and antibacterial by nature – so this property can automatically help in creating a clearer and blemish-free complexion. The temperature of the water also opens the pores and allows them to de-clog and absorb the bacteria-fighting minerals, while the acidity within the water acts as a natural toner. Of course, hot water is naturally cleansing and purifying in itself, removing debris from the surface of the skin and, by enlarging the pores, aids in removing unwanted toxins from within the body. This approach is therefore one of the best ways to detoxify not only the skin, but also our entire system, as part of a complete naturopathic detox program.

Bathing in warm water naturally enhances blood flow and increases the whole body's metabolism. This increases the flow of oxygen to the cells of our body and boosts circulation helping to keep us healthy and full of vitality. Increased blood flow also brings improved nourishment to our vital organs, such as the digestive system and heart. Soaking in thermal water initially increases the heart rate sending blood to the surface of the skin, dispersing extra body heat into the air, but after several minutes the warm water dilates the blood vessels reducing blood flow resistance thus eventually lowering blood pressure. Soaking in a hot bath therefore actually lowers blood pressure, rather than increasing it, as is the case with many physical exercises.

Just taking a regular hot bath can dramatically soothe stiffness of the joints and help ease cramp or muscular tension. The heat and buoyancy of being submerged in hot water is very therapeutic as it helps to reduce the experience of gravity and the weight of our own body. This effect can be enhanced when natural salts with specific minerals, essential oils and clay are added to the bath water. Applying heat packs based on herbal oils or ointments is also a well-known form of therapy for muscular pain or sports injuries, since heat alone fundamentally alleviates tension in tired muscles.

Recent studies conducted in Israel, suggest that bathing can help treat several different kinds of arthritis, including osteoarthritis and rheumatoid arthritis. Those people who took warm baths containing sulphur alongside other therapies, experienced improved strength, better walking ability and less morning stiffness. They also found they had less inflammation, swelling and pain in their joints, particularly in the neck and back. When absorbed through the skin, sulphur has been shown to help alleviate the pain and swelling of arthritic conditions. Mud or clay packs and particularly Dead Sea salt dissolved in a hot bath, also improved symptoms of arthritis, especially when carried out on a daily basis.

Bathing is a particularly beneficial form of treatment for our modern age since it aids all types of conditions exacerbated by stress, including depression, anxiety and nervous exhaustion. With a rich history stretching back thousands of years, thermal bathing does not merely bring relief to those who are ill but plays an equally vital role in preventing the development of stress-related diseases: it is therefore also one of best preventative approaches. Simply soaking in a warm aromatic bath with some essential oils, salts or clay is perhaps one of the most pleasing ways to relax and unwind. Knowing that this is an ancient ritual, which has been practised by all cultures alike as part of a living therapeutic tradition, makes it part of a universal and elemental human experience.

BATHING RECIPES

Most of the recipes here suggest quantities for one bath. But you can always increase the quantities if you would like to make a larger batch by scaling up the proportions and then storing the blend in an airtight container away from direct sunlight. When using mineral salts for bathing, it is recommended that 250 grams (about 8 oz or 1 cup) per day is sufficient for everyday use, but for specific therapeutic effects, such as relieving joint pain, this can be increased to 500 grams (about 1 lb or 2 cups) a day.

For the best hydrotherapy results, it is recommended to add 250 to 500 grams of salt or crystals to the bath water and then soak for at least 15 minutes, where the optimum duration for bathing therapeutically is about 15 to 20 minutes a day over a period of 2 to 3 weeks.

Due to the high concentration of the oils, do not add more than 10 drops (in total) of any combination of essential oils to a bath. Always rest and rehydrate afterwards by drinking a large glass of water or herbal tea!

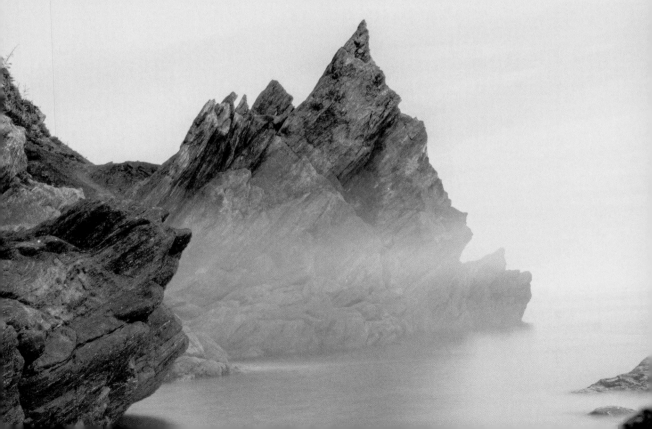

REJUVENATING 'BLUE LAGOON' SOAK

Inspired by the unique Icelandic hot springs, this is a wonderfully relaxing and anti-ageing salt and clay bath. By combining pink Himalayan and Epsom salts with bentonite yellow clay, which mimics the silica mud as found in the famous Blue Lagoon, you can enjoy all the benefits of this truly rejuvenating therapy at home. This treatment is particularly good for mature skin, being rich in silica, which stimulates the production of collagen and helps return tone and elasticity to de-mineralized, dull skin. It also strengthens the hair and nails.

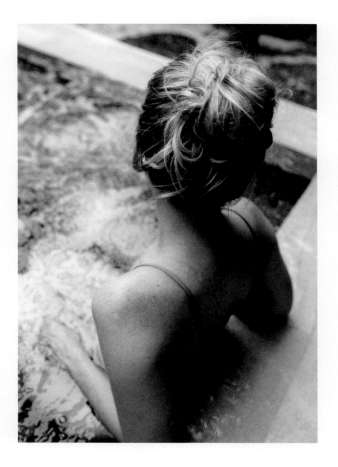

Ingredients:

○   Handful of Himalayan sea salt
○   Handful of Epsom salt
○   Handful of bentonite clay
○   10 drops frankincense essential oil

Directions

Fill a bath with warm water to 30°C (86°F). Add the Himalayan and Epsom salts and agitate the water to ensure they have dissolved. Add the bentonite clay, then add the frankincense essential oil and stir.

Soak in the warm water for up to 20 minutes. Then wrap your entire body in a towel and relax for 15 minutes after bathing to allow for the complete absorption of minerals and nutrients into the skin.

STRESS-RELIEF
SALT SOAK

This relaxing bath blend creates a welcome release from any stress and mental agitation built up over the course of a busy day – it is profoundly soothing both on an emotional and physical level. Vetiver is known as the 'oil of tranquillity'; lavender oil is the classic, sedative remedy that soothes both the senses and psyche; Roman chamomile is a mild yet powerful relaxant oil: the ultimate stress-fix combination!

Ingredients

o   150 grams (5¼ oz) Dead Sea salt
o   100 grams (3½ oz) Epsom salt
o   5 drops lavender essential oil
o   3 drops vetiver essential oil
o   2 drops Roman chamomile
     essential oil

Directions

Fill a bath with hot water to 35°C (95°F). Add the Dead Sea and Epsom salts and agitate the water to ensure they have dissolved. Add the three essential oils and stir.

Soak in the warm water for up to 20 minutes. Then wrap your entire body in a towel and relax for 15 minutes after bathing to allow for the complete absorption of minerals and nutrients into the skin.

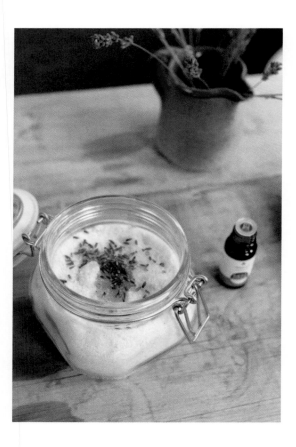

HEALTH TIP

Soaking in hot water initially increases the heart rate, sending blood to the surface and dispersing extra body heat into the air, but after several minutes the warm blood dilates the blood vessels reducing blood flow resistance thus eventually lowering blood pressure.

ACHES + PAINS
SEAWEED SALT SOAK

Rosemary, with its beautiful blue flowers, is known as 'dew of the sea' and is one of the best essential oils for aches, pains, stiffness and general lethargy. Lavender essential oil is valuable for reducing inflammation and joint pain, and for its overall soothing effect. Seaweed is rich in a variety of minerals and helps to relieve aches and pains as well as rheumatism and arthritis. Like rosemary oil, seaweed is also good for the circulation.

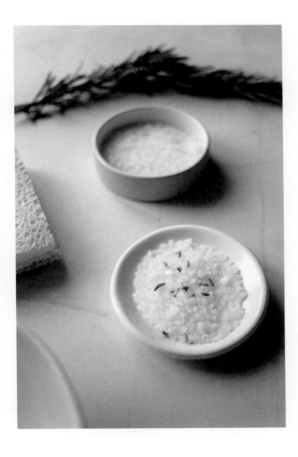

Ingredients

- 150 grams (5¼ oz) Epsom salt
- 100 grams (3½ oz) Dead Sea salt
- 100 grams (3½ oz) coarse sea salt
- 3 tablespoons seaweed powder
- 5 drops rosemary essential oil
- 5 drops lavender essential oil

Directions

Fill a bath with hot water to 35°C (95°F). Add all three salts and ensure they have dissolved by agitating the water. Add the seaweed powder and essential oils and stir.

Soak in the hot water for up to 20 minutes. Then wrap your entire body in a towel and relax for 15 minutes after bathing; to allow for the complete absorption of minerals and nutrients into the skin.

DETOX CORIANDER + CYPRESS SALT SOAK

Coriander and cypress make a dynamic duo when it comes to purification and aiding the body in its natural detoxification process: as diuretic oils they work on both cellulite and water retention.

Ingredients

- ○ 100 grams (3½ oz) Epsom salt
- ○ 100 grams (3½ oz) Himalayan salt
- ○ 50 grams (1¾ oz) Dead Sea salt
- ○ 2 tablespoons seaweed powder
- ○ 2 tablespoons green clay
- ○ 3 drops cypress essential oil
- ○ 3 drops coriander seed essential oil

Directions

Fill a bath with hot water to 35°C (95°F). Add all three salts and ensure they have dissolved by agitating the water. Add the seaweed powder and green clay and stir. Add the essential oils and stir again.

Soak in the warm water for up to 20 minutes. Then wrap your entire body in a towel and relax for 15 minutes after bathing to allow for the complete absorption of minerals and nutrients into the skin.

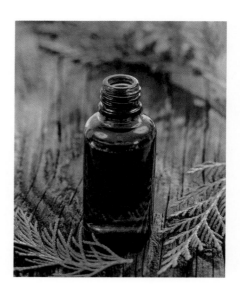

LIFESTYLE TIP

Cypress and coriander are also antispasmodic (pain-relieving) oils, so this is a useful blend for athletes and those training regularly or with active lifestyles. This would also be a useful blend to reset the system after a long flight or if you're feeling a little hungover!

MAGNESIUM-RICH SEAWEED SOAK

Many people are magnesium deficient, so it is beneficial to add Epsom salt to the bath on a regular basis, so the magnesium is absorbed naturally through the skin into the body. It is an especially essential mineral for stressful modern lives as magnesium enables proper nerve and muscle function, supports the metabolism, and eases many common complaints, such as headaches, chronic pain and sleep disorders. Magnesium also helps maintain normal heart rhythms and assists in reducing high blood pressure, palpitations and has been linked to a reduced incidence of conditions, such as heart disease, hypertension and diabetes.

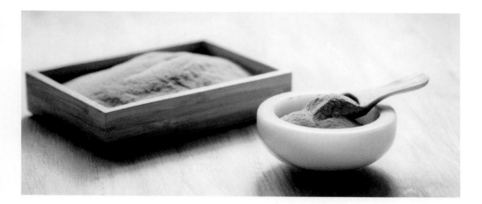

Ingredients

- 250 grams (8 oz) Epsom salt (or magnesium flakes)
- 100 grams (3½ oz) seaweed powder
- 6 drops bergamot essential oil
- 4 drops sandalwood essential oil

Directions

Fill a bath with warm water to 35°C (95°F). Add the Epsom salt and ensure it has dissolved by agitating the water. Add the seaweed powder and stir. Add the essential oils and stir again.

Soak in the warm water for up to 20 minutes. Then wrap your entire body in a towel and relax for 15 minutes after bathing to allow for the complete absorption of minerals and nutrients into the skin.

HEALING + BALANCING BENTONITE CLAY BATH

Bentonite clay is renowned for its therapeutic properties – its high content of silica stimulates the production of protein and collagen, which explains its wide use for anti-ageing treatments. It helps tone and restore elasticity to de-mineralized and dull skin, which makes it great for rejuvenating and healing damaged tissue. Lavender water is healing for the skin and soothing to the psyche while the geranium water has a balancing action – good for periods of emotional or hormonal change, such as during the menopause or menstruation.

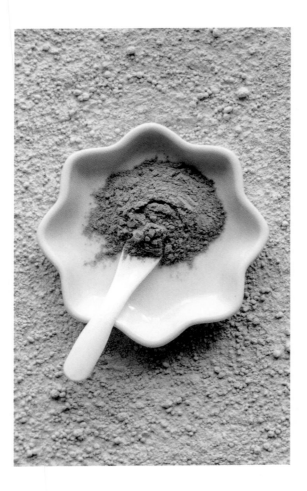

Ingredients

○ 250 grams (8 oz) Dead Sea salt
○ 90 grams (3 oz) bentonite clay
○ 1 tablespoon lavender water
○ 1 tablespoon geranium water

Directions

Fill a bath with warm water to 35°C (95°F). Add the Dead Sea salt and ensure it has dissolved by agitating the water.

Pour the clay into a bowl, adding the lavender and geranium waters slowly to create a paste. Stir for a few minutes until combined. Once ready, add the mixture to the freshly run warm bath. Agitate the water with your hand or use a wooden spoon to mix.

Soak for up to 20 minutes. Then wrap your entire body in a towel and relax for 15 minutes after bathing to allow for the complete absorption of minerals and nutrients into the skin.

IMMUNE SUPPORT AROMATIC BATH OIL

I don't like to use vegetable oils in the bath a great deal as it can make the sides of the bath slippery, which can be dangerous, especially for the elderly. But here the essential oils are mixed first with a base oil to ensure they are thoroughly blended before adding a little to the bath water. Rosemary is one of my favourite herbs for combatting contagious infections, especially respiratory conditions, and by soaking in a hot bath this effectively is the same as carrying out a steam inhalation. Fragonia oil supports the immune system and has powerful bactericidal, antiseptic, anti-inflammatory and antimicrobial activity, much like tea tree oil, but is much milder on the skin with a pleasing citrus-like scent.

Ingredients

o   50 ml (1¾ fl oz) light coconut oil
o   20 drops rosemary essential oil
o   15 drops fragonia essential oil
o   5 drops black pepper essential oil
o   5 drops of bergamot essential oil
o   5 drops myrtle essential oil

Directions

Add the light coconut oil to a clean 60-ml (2-fl oz) tinted glass bottle with a pipette top. Add the drops of essential oils carefully one by one. Place the lid on and give the bottle a good shake.

To use, add 2 pipettes to a freshly run bath, with water at a temperature of 35°C (95°F), and stir well. Soak in the tub for up to 20 minutes.

LIFESTYLE TIP

The oil will cling to your skin when you step out of the bath, but remember to remove any oily residue from the tub.

ROMANTIC RITUAL FLORAL BATH

This is a recipe for a romantic candle-lit bathing experience with the option of adding fresh flower petals to the bath for their delightful aesthetic effect. The original method for producing rose water was simply to float scented rose petals in warm water until it was saturated with their scent, then the precious rose water was filtered off. The coconut powder softens the skin.

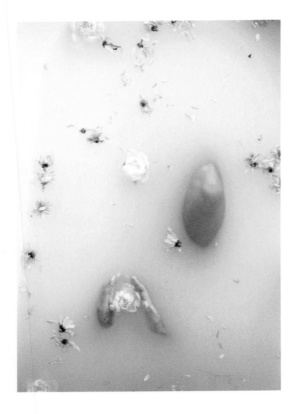

Ingredients

o   150 grams (5¼ oz) coconut milk powder
o   1 tablespoon rosehip powder
o   2 drops rose essential oil
o   2 drops jasmine essential oil
o   2 drops ylang ylang essential oil
o   Handful of fresh flower petals, such as rose, borage or chamomile (optional)

Directions

Fill a bath with hot water to 35°C (95°F). Add the coconut milk and rosehip powder to the water. Add all the essential oils. Light a candle and float some fresh petals on the surface of the water, if using.

Soak in the warm water for up to 20 minutes. Then wrap your entire body in a towel and relax for 15 minutes after bathing to allow for the complete absorption of minerals and nutrients into the skin.

VARIATION

It is possible to also make your own rosehip powder at home by collecting rosehips then drying them and finally whizzing them in a blender.

RHASSOUL + ROSEHIP FOR MATURE SKIN

Rhassoul clay is a fine, red clay from Morocco that has been used for centuries in skincare. When added to a warm bath, it turns the water a soft ruby colour. It is much gentler than many other clays and is typically recommended for sensitive and mature skin types. It gently stimulates blood circulation, bringing fresh nutrients to the tissues. Rosehip seed oil is rich in retinoic acid found in vitamin A, which can help eliminate fine lines, while the antioxidants and omega fatty acids also protect cells from premature ageing.

Ingredients

○ 60 grams (2 oz) rhassoul clay
○ 1 tablespoon rosehip seed oil
○ Sprinkle of fresh or dried rose petals (optional)

Directions

Pour the rhassoul clay to a bowl, adding the rosehip seed oil slowly, stirring to create a paste. Once ready, add the mix to a freshly run warm bath. Agitate the water with your hand or using a wooden spoon to mix. Sprinkle the rose petals into the tub, if using. Soak for up to 20 minutes.

VARIATION

For a bactericidal action, add up to 10 drops of fragonia essential oil to the water.

MOISTURIZING BATH OIL FOR DRY SKIN

This moisturizing bath oil makes an indulgent treat for promoting silky-soft skin and is excellent for dry, dehydrated and sun-damaged skin. You can also apply this oil blend directly to dry skin, especially reddish areas, following a day in the sun. Lavender oil soothes burned skin plus relaxes the senses and psyche; myrrh is an oleo-gum resin with profound and ancient healing qualities; frankincense is a well-known rejuvenating agent through increasing cellular regeneration.

Ingredients

○ 50 ml (1¾ fl oz) light coconut oil
○ 15 drops lavender essential oil
○ 15 drops frankincense essential oil
○ 10 drops myrrh essential oil

Directions

Add the light coconut oil to a clean 60-ml (2-fl oz) tinted glass bottle with a pipette top or atomizer lid for ease of use. Add the essential oils one by one. Place the lid on and shake.

To use, add 2 pipettes or 4 spritzes to a freshly run warm bath. Soak for up to 20 minutes.

LIFESTYLE TIP

Spray this oil directly on the skin after bathing or showering to lock in moisture.

GORGEOUS GREEN
BATH FOR OILY SKIN

French green clay has a light green tone when dry and turns a rich gorgeous green colour when it is added to the bath water. Like seaweed, it is very rich in minerals, mainly silica, while the verdant colour comes from decomposed ancient plant matter within the clay. Green clay comes from rich volcanic soils (originally from France) where it is famous for its excellent healing action alongside deep detoxification and purification properties. It is especially suited to oily skin having many therapeutic applications. It deeply cleans the skin, removing the dead surface cells and toxins, while its high absorption properties remove grease and help tighten the skin, reducing the look of prominent pores and blackheads.

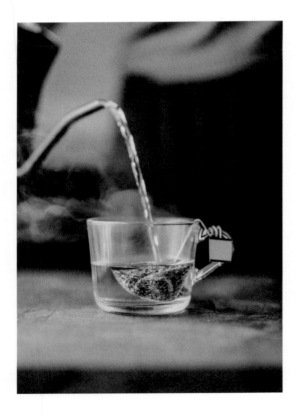

Ingredients

o   60 grams (2 oz) green clay
o   2 tablespoons seaweed powder
o   I cup brewed green tea
    (hot or cold)

Directions

Pour the green clay and seaweed powder into a bowl, adding the green tea slowly to create a paste while mixing with a wooden spoon. Stir for a few minutes until combined. Once ready, add the mixture to a freshly run warm bath. Agitate the water with your hand or use a wooden spoon to mix.

Soak for up to 20 minutes.

LUXURIOUS COCONUT MILK BATH FOR SUPER SOFT SKIN

Cleopatra was renowned for bathing in donkey's milk and honey to keep her skin looking youthful and luxuriously soft and supple. Using any form of dairy milk in the bath and on the skin, however, is not ideal as once the milk dries out it develops an unpleasant odour. This recipe using coconut milk is an innovative way I have discovered to enjoy the benefits. Once added to the bath water, the coconut milk turns a milky-white colour, making the bath water feel beautifully soft and gentle on the skin. The coconut milk also nourishes, softens and hydrates skin. In addition to the honey, I have added a little rose oil here, for a truly luxurious effect.

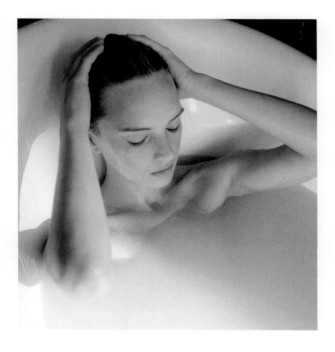

Ingredients

- 100 ml (3½ fl oz) light coconut milk
- 1 tablespoon runny honey
- 10 drops rose maroc 5 per cent essential oil (or 2 drops wild rose or rose otto)

Directions

Fill a bath with warm water to 35°C (95°F). Add the coconut milk and agitate the water to make sure it is well mixed. Add the honey beneath the running hot tap to ensure it dissolves fully. Add the rose essential oil and stir.

Soak in the warm water for up to 20 minutes. Then wrap your entire body in a towel and relax for 15 minutes to allow for the complete absorption of oils and nutrients into the skin.

SOOTHING OAT SOAK FOR IRRITATED SKIN

Oats have outstanding benefits for the skin, particularly when it comes to dry, itchy skin and flare-ups of conditions such as eczema, dermatitis and psoriasis. Oats contain proteins, vitamin E, betaglucan, and carbohydrates hence why they make a great snack for the skin too! Oats have excellent emollient and antioxidant properties that work to reduce inflammation and irritation when added to the bath, while locking in moisture, making the skin feel supple, soft and deeply soothed. For highly sensitive skins, bathing in powdered oatmeal alone is recommended, but do a patch test first if you wish to add the essential oils to the bath.

Ingredients

- 100 grams (3½ oz) rolled oats or colloidal oatmeal
- 1 cup calendula herbal tea
- 4 drops lavender essential oil
- 4 drops myrrh essential oil
- 2 drops German chamomile essential oil
- 2 drops rose maroc 5 per cent essential oil

Directions

Put the dry rolled oats into a blender and whizz until powdered, for approximately 2 minutes. You can blend the oats in larger batches and store in a container in a cool, dry cupboard to use as needed.

Add 1 cup of ground oats or colloidal oatmeal to a freshly run warm bath. Add the calendula infusion. Add the essential oils – no more than 10 drops in total.

Soak in the bath for up to 20 minutes.

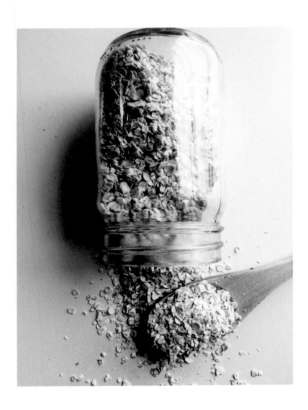

VARIATION

You can also add optional extras, such as an infusion of calendula flowers or a few drops each of the following essential oils – lavender, rose, chamomile and myrrh – but add no more than 10 drops in total.

KAOLIN, OAT + ALOE FOR SENSITIVE SKIN

Kaolin or white clay has a neutral pH for the skin, so this clay is recommended for all types of skin but especially sensitive skin. The texture of white clay is very fine and soft, and it has a gentle natural whitening action on the skin when used in the bath and in body treatments. It is not as absorbent as other clays, making it suitable for skin that tends to be drier or more sensitive. Because it has a pH value similar to the skin, white clay is especially suited to delicate skin as well as for use as a natural baby powder – an ideal substitute to talcs.

Ingredients

- 60 grams (2 oz) kaolin/white clay
- 2 tablespoons finely ground oats
- 2 tablespoons aloe vera water or gel

Directions

Pour the kaolin clay and oats into a bowl, adding the aloe vera slowly to create a paste. Stir for a few minutes until combined.

Once ready, add the mixture to a freshly run warm bath. Agitate the water with your hand or using a wooden spoon to mix.

Soak for up to 15 minutes.

CHILDREN'S OAT BATH FOR DELICATE SKIN

My mother Kerttu was a great fan of using colloidal oatmeal or oat milk in the bath for soothing delicate or irritated skin, for treating children's rashes and to help combat itchy complaints, such as heat rash and chickenpox. Only recently researchers have discovered that a phenolic alkaloid called avenanthramide in the oats is responsible for soothing the skin.

Ingredients

- 100 grams (3½ oz) colloidal oatmeal or 100 ml (3½ fl oz) oat milk
- Fresh or dried lavender tops, rose petals or chamomile flowers (or others of your choice)

Directions

Add the oatmeal (or oat milk) to a freshly run warm bath. Add a handful of fresh or dried herbs, such as lavender, chamomile or rose petals, loose or secured in a bath sachet.

Soak in the bath for 5 to 10 minutes – children should not soak for too long due to their delicate skin.

HEALTH TIP

Avoid using essential oils in the bath for very young children; instead add fresh flowers or herbs.

HERB + FLOWER BATH

Herbs and flowers picked from the garden can be enjoyed in the bath by simply making the flower heads or leafy sprigs into a bunch and then tying them around the hot tap using ribbon or string. When you are using herbs in this way, it can be also be helpful to create a re-usable bath sachet using a square of muslin or linen cloth or a pre-made drawstring bag to contain the herbs, so there's no tidying up or removing bits of herbs and flowers from the bathtub afterwards.

Ingredients

Here are a few suggestions for fresh flowers and herbs to collect.

o   Dry skin: chamomile, lavender, marigold
o   Aches and pains: lavender, rosemary, peppermint
o   Sleep: lemon balm, chamomile, lavender
o   Refreshing: lemon verbena, fennel, peppermint

Directions

Strip the flowers and leaves from your collected herbs and flowers. Mix 1 tablespoon of each herb you are using in a small bowl. Place on a pre-cut 20-cm (8-in) muslin square or, alternatively, into a ready-made drawstring linen or muslin bag. Tie some string or ribbon around to secure the herbs inside.

To use, tie around the hot tap while you are running the bath or simply drop the sachet into the bath water. Float flower heads on the surface of the water for a luxurious experience. Soak in the floral and herbal infusion for 10 to 15 minutes.

LIFESTYLE TIP

Homemade bath sachets stuffed with aromatic herbs also make lovely gifts. You can experiment with different herb and flower combinations; children especially love to pick flowers and herbs to add to their bath in this way.

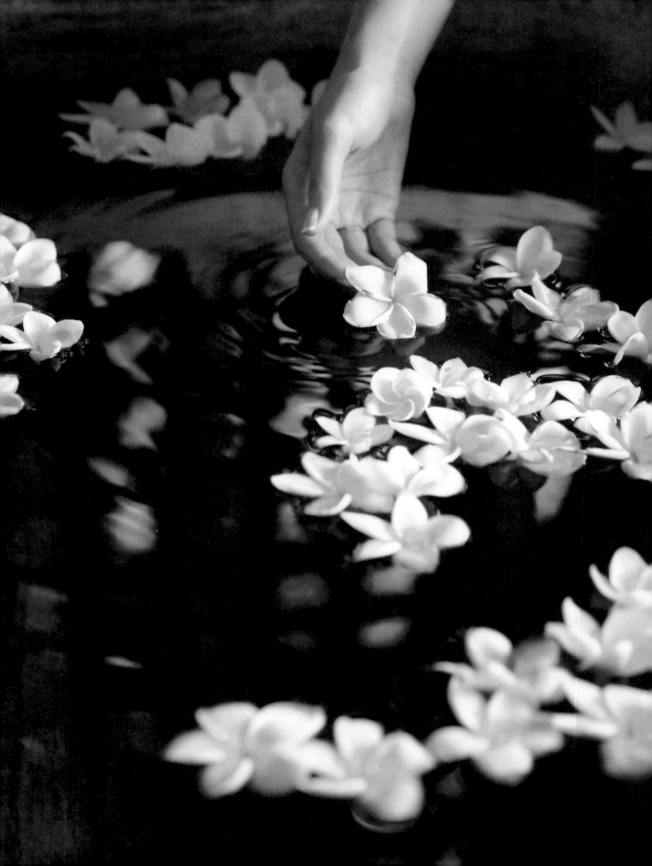

SIMPLE HERBAL
HAND SOAK

This is a simple recipe for keeping your hands and nails looking healthy and helping to get rid of any unsightly cuts or infections. It can be made using either fresh herbs gathered from the garden or using the essential oils extracted from the same plants. Peppermint, rosemary and lavender is a lovely combination for the hands to cleanse, purify and refresh. Jojoba oil is a superb moisturizing agent and myrrh oil is added for its healing properties.

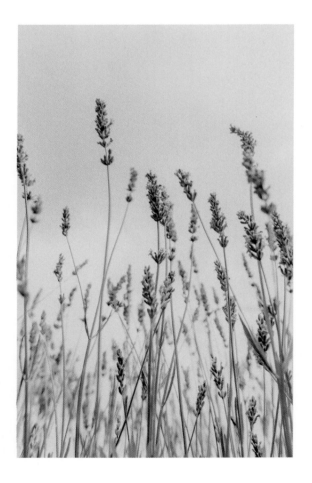

Ingredients

o   2 drops rosemary essential oil
    (or a sprig of the fresh herb)
o   2 drops lavender essential oil
    (or a sprig of the fresh herb)
o   2 drops peppermint essential oil
    (or a sprig of the fresh herb)
o   1 drop myrrh essential oil
o   1 teaspoon jojoba oil

Directions

Fill a shallow bowl or basin to the brim with hot water. If using fresh herbs, add these to the water immediately for their aromatic effects. Add the myrrh oil plus any other essential oils to the jojoba oil and then add this to the bowl.

Place your hands in the aromatic hot water, gently massaging the oils and herbs into your palms, fingers and cuticles, and soak your hands for 10 to 15 minutes while relaxing.

SOOTHING FOOT SOAK

Your feet work extremely hard for you every day and this salt soak is best enjoyed at the end of a busy day or at a weekend as part of a 'home spa' session. This recipe, which is nourishing and moisturizing, also helps deal with foot conditions such as dry cracked skin, athlete's foot and fungal nail infections.

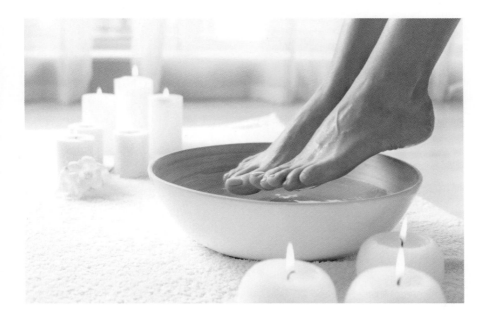

Ingredients

- o   150 grams (5¼ oz) Epsom salt
- o   2 drops eucalyptus essential oil
- o   2 drops lavender essential oil
- o   2 drops bergamot essential oil
- o   1 teaspoon argan oil

Directions

Fill a shallow bowl to the brim with hot water. Add the Epsom salt and ensure it has dissolved by agitating the water. Add all the essential oils to the argan oil and mix, then add this blend to the water and stir well again.

Soak your feet in the aromatic water for 10 to 15 minutes while relaxing.

MULTIPURPOSE CASTILE SOAP

This is a simple soap recipe that can be enjoyed in the bath, shower or as a daily hand wash, including for sensitive skin. Castile soap is a 100 per cent natural product, which makes an excellent body cleanser, hand wash, shampoo and laundry detergent as it has a mild pH that will not dry out the skin. To add a gentle exfoliation to your soap, add jojoba beads, which do not irritate the skin. Extracted from the waxes of the jojoba plant, they are entirely natural and biodegradable. Palmarosa, a type of grass with gently purifying properties, and chamomile help soothe inflammation and irritations, such as eczema and psoriasis, and lavender forms a gentle synergy that is both bactericidal and antiseptic.

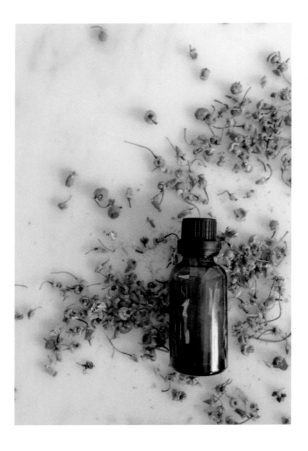

Ingredients

o   95 ml (3¼ fl oz) unscented liquid Castile soap
o   1 teaspoon vegetable glycerine
o   2 teaspoons jojoba oil
o   1 teaspoon jojoba beads (optional)
o   10 drops palmarosa essential oil
o   10 drops lavender essential oil
o   10 drops German chamomile essential oil

Directions

Add the Castile soap, vegetable glycerine and jojoba oil to a clean 100-ml (3½-fl oz) tinted glass bottle with a pump top. Add the essential oils one by one. Add the jojoba beads, if using. Place the lid on the bottle and shake vigorously.

The soap is ready to use immediately, applying to dry or damp skin and rinsing off in the bath, shower or sink.

SEA SALT HAND SCRUB

A sea salt scrub is an excellent way to lift dirt and debris after time spent in the garden or doing DIY projects around the house; it can remove caked-on dirt and help to break down any grease from household products, paint and ink. Plus, it has the added benefit of being antiseptic and antibacterial, disinfecting any cuts and scrapes you might have sustained. Apricot kernel oil is a lovely gentle nourishing carrier oil, well suited to sensitive or irritated skin – it also supports the protective barrier of the skin while improving elasticity and texture. Lavender and lemon essential oils make a refreshing combination for the skin and senses, and both are antibacterial and antiseptic.

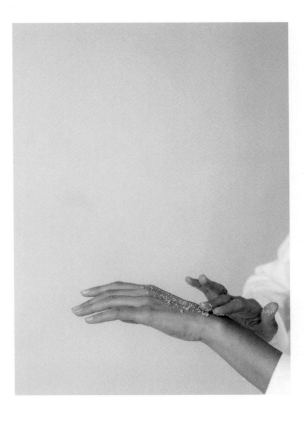

Ingredients

- o   3 tablespoons sea salt
- o   1 tablespoon apricot kernel oil
- o   2 drops lavender essential oil
- o   2 drops lemon essential oil
- o   Handful of fresh lemon balm leaves (optional)

Directions

Add the salt to a bowl first, then slowly add the apricot kernel oil to create a paste, stirring with a wooden spoon. Add the essential oils and stir again. Add finely chopped lemon balm leaves, if using.

Once ready, apply to dry or slightly damp hands by rubbing gently using a circulation motion. To finish, simply rinse off, or repeat if needed.

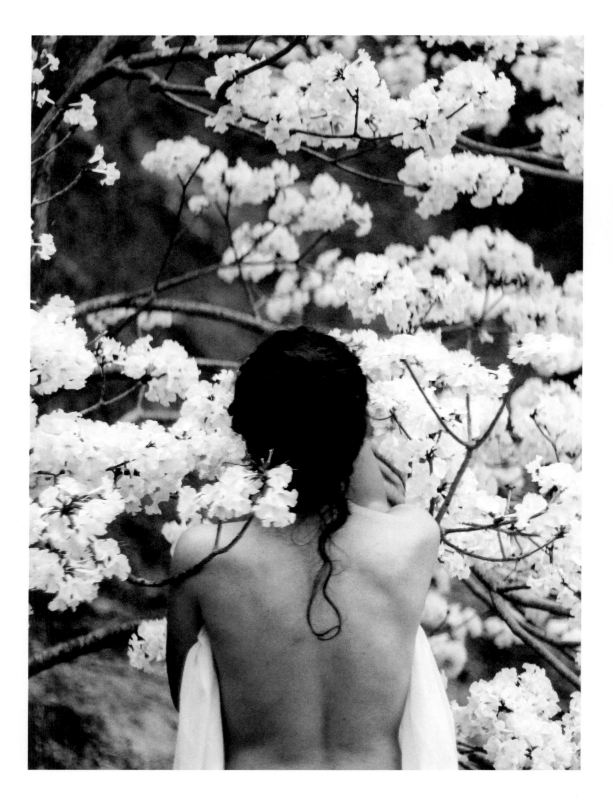

'Massage is the oldest known form of therapy; it has been indicated for restoration of physical health and relief of psychological stress throughout history and in most cultures.'

JENNIFER PEACE RHIND, *ESSENTIAL OILS*

2 + BODY

Massage + Body Treatments

The healing powers of massage have been practiced since ancient times and have benefits that go far beyond the realm of the physical. We instinctively respond to human touch from birth, and the importance of skin-to-skin contact represents a vital ingredient in our overall sense of wellbeing and self-esteem. Massage is therefore a natural and intrinsic part of the naturopathic traditions: Hippocrates recommended a daily aromatic bath and a fragrant massage as a preventative treatment for both our mind and body. On a psychological level, massage helps us to slow down, de-stress and become more aware and present in the moment. Research has also shown that massage releases the hormone serotonin that enhances the body and mind 'feel good' state. Massage also increases delta wave frequency in our brains, which is closely associated with a deep sense of relaxation, restfulness and sleep. The benefits of massage for pre-natal and post-natal women as well as for babies and children can't be overemphasized because of the profoundly nurturing aspect of this type of natural therapy.

On a physical level, massage improves blood circulation, which delivers oxygen and nutrients to the cells, while simultaneously stimulating the lymphatic system that carries away the body's waste products. Massage is well known as an aid in limbering up the body before sporting activities and professional athletes regularly use massage to ease muscular tension and cramps after an event. Massage therapy can also help with pain management in chronic conditions like arthritis, sciatica and muscle spasms, especially in combination with other natural treatments, such as salt and mineral baths. In addition, techniques like lymphatic drainage and deep tissue bodywork can help keep the body in shape. When combined with other approaches, such as therapeutic mud and salt treatments, this can further help eliminate dead skin cells, eliminate toxins and decrease cellulite.

In terms of overall skincare, massage gently helps exfoliate the skin, while promoting cellular renovation, refining the pores and giving the skin a uniform appearance. Massage plays a central role in the art of aromatherapy, where the main botanical oils or carrier oils, such as sweet almond oil, act as the perfect base for specific essential oils to be applied to the skin. The skin is the body's largest organ of our body and promoting good circulation via massage helps rid the body of harmful substances. Massage also enhances the secretion of natural oils, which moisturize and lubricate the skin, helping to keep it healthy and supple. Increased blood flow to the outer layers of the skin transports oxygen to the surface blood bringing nutrients to the new cells while the lymph fluid flowing away from the skin carries impurities with it. Quite apart from the nurturing effects of touch, some of the direct benefits of aromatherapy massage are that it increases the circulation, removes dead cells from the outer dermis and helps eliminate toxins from the body.

Our skin absorbs over 70 per cent of whatever it is exposed to, including pollution, so it is vital that at night we ensure our pores are allowed to breathe freely. Cleansing our bodies regularly is therefore a key factor in keeping our skin looking fresh and radiant – the night is also the ideal time for our skin to absorb nutrient-rich oils using self-massage. Ideally, massage oils are best applied to warm skin to encourage absorption, such as after a hot bath or shower. Do not be afraid to use your intuition in deciding which type of massage strokes to use – some conditions clearly require a more vigorous approach, while others ask for a gentle touch. Facial massage should also always be carried out with great sensitivity. Avoid dragging on the skin, especially around the eyes, and always direct stokes upwards and outwards. Likewise, massage for children and babies should always be done very gently using specifically chosen oils.

Applying body and facial oils is a valuable way to use self-massage as part of a daily skincare routine. For a whole body pamper, first exfoliate using vigorous strokes from the feet upwards with a natural bristle brush to cleanse the skin thoroughly. Massage your entire body with small circular movements using a light carrier oil, such as sweet almond oil or grapeseed oil, to boost the metabolism. Then step under a warm shower and gently rub your skin down using a natural flannel or bath mitt. In this case, the steam and prior exfoliating rub will aid the absorption of the natural oils. Finally, apply an aromatic body oil suited to your skin type to promote a silky-smooth skin. Applying an oil prior to showering can also be a valuable technique if you have very dry or sensitive skin since the oil acts as protection or barrier against the heat.

Quite apart from being the ideal carriers for massage with essential oils, many botanical or vegetable oils have outstanding skincare and hair-conditioning qualities. For example, rosehip seed oil is one of the most useful oils for the skin. Packed full of vitamins, antioxidants and essential fatty acids, rosehip seed oil is a rich source of vitamin C. This makes it a primary choice for skin regeneration and nutrition together with providing a range of anti-ageing benefits. It stimulates skin cell growth and renewal, promotes collagen production, while helping to maintain the elasticity of the tissue, thus helping it to stay soft, smooth and young looking. Above all, rosehip seed oil can protect skin cells from premature ageing when used regularly and can act as a preventive measure against stretch marks or long-term scarring. Rosehip seed oil's anti-ageing properties combined with its super-light and non-greasy texture make it the ideal component in facial oils. It also helps to keep the skin in optimum health when used as a 'booster' active ingredient in a body or massage oil blend.

Applying a specially formulated aromatic body oil to the skin on a daily basis after showering or bathing is the optimum way to ensure that all the skin remains healthy. Body oils can also be adapted to specific conditions – for example, cellulite or fatty deposits can be tackled by massaging the area with blends using lightweight carrier oils, such coconut or jojoba oil, combined with essential oils having detoxifying and purifying qualities, such as fennel seed. Regions of very dry skin on the body, such as on the feet or elbows, can be treated using richly nourishing oils, like avocado oil, combined with the healing qualities of myrrh essential oil. Lips can be nourished, moisturized

and prevented from drying or cracking using natural balms and salves. By combining aromatic oils with other treatments, such as exfoliating rubs and masks, we can be sure that we are looking after our skin in the best way possible. Like body or massage oils, these treatments can be adapted to skin type and needs, using active ingredients such as clay, charcoal, salt, herbs and butters.

It is important to remember that our hands and feet, including our nails, also need some TLC. I like to use nourishing butters, such shea butter or cocoa butter, combined with specific essential oil, on my hands and feet. Applying rich butters helps to keep the nails and cuticles in good condition, while the addition of an essential oil can help heal and eliminate any cuts or infections on our hands or feet. In all cases, it is good to give our nails a break from using nail varnish regularly and instead to treat them using moisturizing oils and balms. Nail biting is also naturally reduced if you take the time to look after your fingernails, so they look nice to start with!

A foot bath followed by a foot massage is perhaps one of the most underestimated luxuries of life. This is not only a profoundly relaxing experience, especially after a tiring day on your feet, but also serves to help eliminate common foot or nail conditions, such as athlete's foot or corns. It is worth remembering that feet and hands, like ears, have pressure points which connect to all the internal organs of the body, so massaging any of these areas can simultaneously support the whole system.

Looking after our hair can also be a pleasurable and rewarding experience since our hair says a lot about how we feel about ourselves. The condition of the hair is also a good indicator of the overall state of health and well-being. Hair and nails are always the last in line to receive nutrients, so we need to eat a well-balanced diet and have a healthy lifestyle if we want to have luscious, shiny hair. Lack of sleep, stress, smoking and too much alcohol will also result in dull, lifeless hair and sometimes even in hair loss. The first step towards healthy hair is to improve overall lifestyle and to replace harsh shampoos and chemical treatments with natural alternatives.

Many commercial shampoos contain sodium laurel sulphate, a scalp irritant, so it is important to use a shampoo that is sulphate free. Like the skin, our hair is naturally acidic, so frequent washing with an alkaline shampoo will upset the PH acid balance and strip the hair of its natural oils. Only shampoo your hair when it really needs it and use lukewarm water for washing it and cold water for the final rinse. It is also important to rinse the hair well after using any shampoo to avoid a build-up of residue on the scalp. By simply ceasing to use harsh shampoos, many conditions such as dandruff and even hair loss, will start to improve. It is also beneficial to keep the use of a hairdryer to a minimum to avoid hair damage and scalp problems: instead, towel dry your hair

until it's 80 per cent dry, then use a low heat to blow dry it, if required.

All types of hair benefit from being treated with essential oils, alongside health-enhancing conditioners. For example, for hair loss, avoid intense heat or chemical treatments and wear a hat if it's sunny, as most hair loss problems start with damage to the scalp and roots of the hair. The scalp is made of cells which continually work their way to the surface and the dead cells need to be removed for the scalp to be healthy. If the follicles become blocked by sebum or by dead skin, for example, it may even result in the hair not growing at all! Massaging the head and scalp with natural oils promotes circulation and encourages hair growth, and reduces dry skin and dandruff. For greasy hair, avoid very hot water while shampooing as this further stimulates the sebaceous glands. Mud is also great for oily scalps, as is any kind of clay or kaolin powder. These help to tackle excess oil and remove toxins. Massaging a mud-based mask into the scalp once a week will help to eliminate grease.

Each week, find the time for a home spa session – to look after the body and to condition nails and hair. Jojoba oil is one of the best all-round conditioning treatments as it lubricates and softens the skin, plus it improves hair quality by giving it shine, restores damaged hair shafts and also nourishes the scalp. Specific treatments for the body and for all hair types, including for beards, can be found in the recipe section.

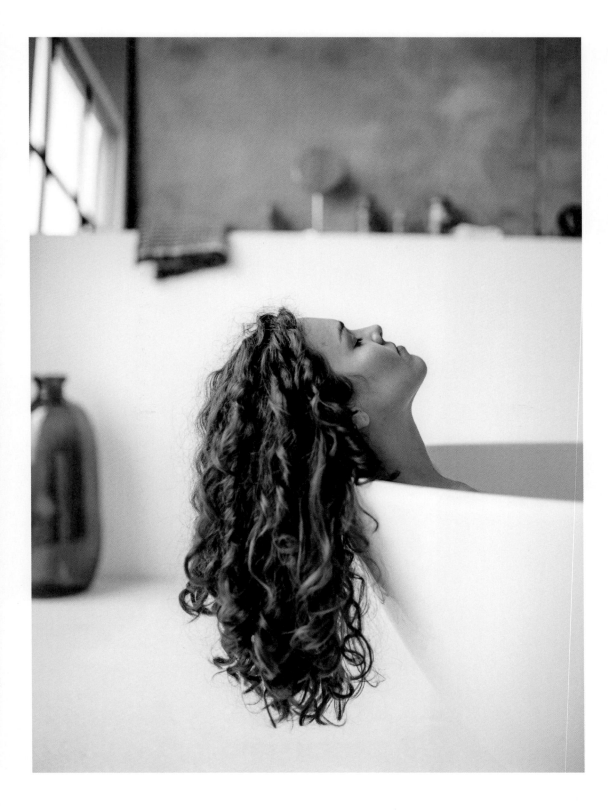

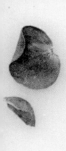

BODY RECIPES

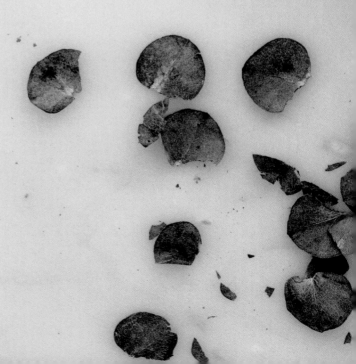

When you are preparing recipes for the body and hair, this often involves larger quantities of ingredients than for the bath, face, first aid or for perfume blends. So it is good to start with a clean table, mixing bowls, a wooden spoon (do not use a metal spoon as this may react with the minerals in the salt or clays), clean tinted bottles and jars with tight-fitting lids, as well as all the ingredients you want to use laid out in front of you, so you are well prepared. You will also need glass measuring beakers, glass stirring rods and funnels to ensure you are able to follow the recipes precisely. It can be nice to collect decorative jars and bottles to make your creations look pleasing – and of course it is best to label everything clearly immediately, including the date you made it, so you remember when you need to use it by. For single-use masks or scrubs, this is not important, but once you start making up body or massage oils in larger quantities, then you will need to be aware of their shelf life.

The benefit of using coconut oil or jojoba oil as the base oil is that they are both very stable – this means they do not deteriorate over time. Most of the body treatments recommended here are stable for at least 6 months unless otherwise stated, such as single-use recipes.

SLIMMING SALT SCRUB

Exfoliating the whole body with an invigorating salt scrub brings blood to the surface of the skin, increasing the circulation and metabolism, while at the same time making the skin feel soft and smooth. The addition of stimulating aromatic oils in the recipe helps break down any fatty deposits or cellulite and further enhances the detoxifying effects.

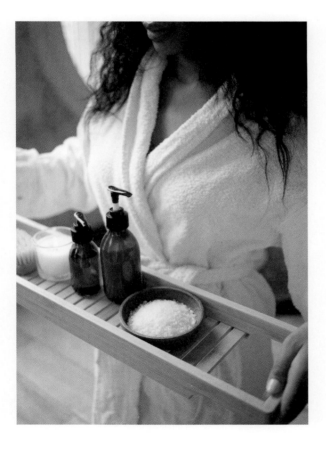

Ingredients

- 100 grams (3½ oz) Epsom salt
- 100 ml (3½ fl oz) jojoba oil
- 10 drops juniper essential oil
- 10 drops rosemary essential oil
- 10 drops grapefruit essential oil

Directions

Add the Epsom salt to a large clean glass jar with a tight-fitting lid. Pour in the jojoba oil. Add all the essential oils one by one and stir well. Secure the lid of the jar tightly.

Allow to infuse for a week, shaking occasionally.

To use, rub the skin vigorously all over with a handful of the salt scrub for 5 to 10 minutes. Rinse clean while standing in the bath or shower.

REGENERATIVE COFFEE + SUGAR SCRUB

The main ingredients in this recipe can be found in your kitchen cupboard. Brown sugar has an effective skin regenerative action and helps rehydrate the skin, while the glycolic acid present helps diminish scars and can control melanin formation, thus helping to prevent dark age spots from developing. Coffee is naturally full of antioxidants and has an excellent exfoliating action when applied to the skin. This recipe makes enough for one full body scrub.

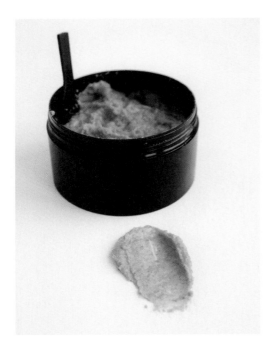

Ingredients

○ 3 tablespoons used coffee grounds
○ 3 tablespoons brown sugar
○ 1 teaspoon sweet almond oil.
○ 1 tablespoon raw runny honey
○ 2 drops rosemary essential oil
○ 2 drops mandarin essential oil
○ 2 drops clary sage essential oil

Directions

Mix all the ingredients together in a bowl in the order described above and stir until all the items are combined well. Test a bit of the mixture by rubbing it onto your hands to check the consistency and so that you can feel the grain of the scrub on the skin.

To use, apply in a circular motion onto dry or damp skin, starting from the feet upwards towards the neck, but not including the face. Rinse off in the bath or shower after about 5 minutes.

LIFESTYLE TIP

You can also recycle your spent coffee grounds in a scrub simply by rubbing them in a circular motion on the skin, before rinsing off in the bath or shower.

HEALING JOJOBA + HONEY BODY POLISH

This formulation is aimed at making the skin of your whole body soft and super smooth. The salt used is fine grain, so rather than providing exfoliation, this is more like a body polish to help make the skin texture uniform and even. The addition of honey, mud and frankincense essential oil also ensures the skin is nourished and replenished with vital minerals. This recipe makes just enough for one full body treatment.

Ingredients

- 2 teaspoons jojoba oil
- 3 tablespoons fine sea salt
- 3 tablespoons jojoba beads
- 1 tablespoon raw honey
- 1 tablespoon kaolin/white clay
- 2 drops frankincense essential oil

Directions

Mix all the ingredients together in a bowl with a wooden spoon in the order described above. Test a bit of the blend by rubbing it onto your hands to check the consistency has a thick grainy texture and to ensure all the ingredients are combined well.

To use, apply in a circular motion onto dry or damp skin, starting from the feet upwards and finishing with the neck, but avoiding the face. Leave on for 5 minutes before rinsing off in the bath or shower.

DETOXIFYING BODY MASK

Fuller's earth clay has very strong oil absorbing abilities and, because of this, it is recommended for those with very oily skin as well as for purification and detox purposes. The dry clay has a slightly earthy scent and a fine, pale powdery texture, making it easy to mix with liquids. It is suitable for normal to oily skin and scalps, but it is not suited to those with very dry skin. Green clay is healing and draws out impurities from the body; honey ensures the skin remains hydrated; witch hazel is astringent and antiseptic. This recipe is for a single-use quantity.

Ingredients

- 50 grams (1¾ oz) Fuller's earth
- 50 grams (1¾ oz) green clay
- 1 tablespoon runny honey
- 3 drops eucalyptus essential oil
- 3 drops petitgrain essential oil
- 1–2 tablespoons witch hazel water

Directions

Put the two clays in a mixing bowl and add the honey and essential oils. Mix well with a wooden spoon to combine. Add the witch hazel slowly, taking care the mixture remains a paste and does not become too thin.

To use, apply the mask to the feet first, then move up the rest of the body, finishing with the hands and neck. Avoid the face. Leave on for 15 to 20 minutes before rinsing off with warm water.

MOROCCAN CLARIFYING BODY MASK

Rhassoul red clay has been in use for over 1,400 years! It was formed under the Atlas Mountains in Morocco – its name means 'the mountain of the washer' in Arabic. Women have long prized its protective, regenerative and healing properties, while its active compounds are quickly absorbed into the skin, leaving it soft and smooth. Due to its fine texture and mobility when mixed with liquids, it makes an excellent ingredient for body masks suited to all skin types. Research shows that a single use of rhassoul clay can improve skin firmness by 24 per cent, skin clarity by 68 per cent and reduce dryness by as much as 79 per cent and flakiness by 41 per cent. When applied to the skin, it removes dead cells and excess sebum, which are major contributors to acne – it is also employed as part of the traditional hammam bathing rituals. Make a fresh batch for each use.

Ingredients

- 50 grams (1¾ oz) dried rose petals
- 100 grams (3½ oz) rhassoul clay
- ½ teaspoon argan oil
- ½ teaspoon rose flower water
- 2 drops neroli essential oil
- 2 drops jasmine essential oil
- 2 drops geranium essential oil

Directions

Grind the rose petals in a food processor, blender or using a pestle and mortar. Add the ground petals to the rhassoul clay in a bowl. Add the argan oil slowly and stir with a wooden spoon, until it forms a thick paste. Add the rose flower water slowly and stir with a spoon, ensuring the mix stays paste-like and not too watery. Add the essential oils last and stir well to combine everything together.

To use, apply the mask to the feet first then move up the rest of the body, doing the hands, neck and face last – being careful to keep it away from the eyes. Leave on for 10 to 20 minutes until the mask has completely dried and the skin feels tight. Rinse off with warm water in the bath or shower.

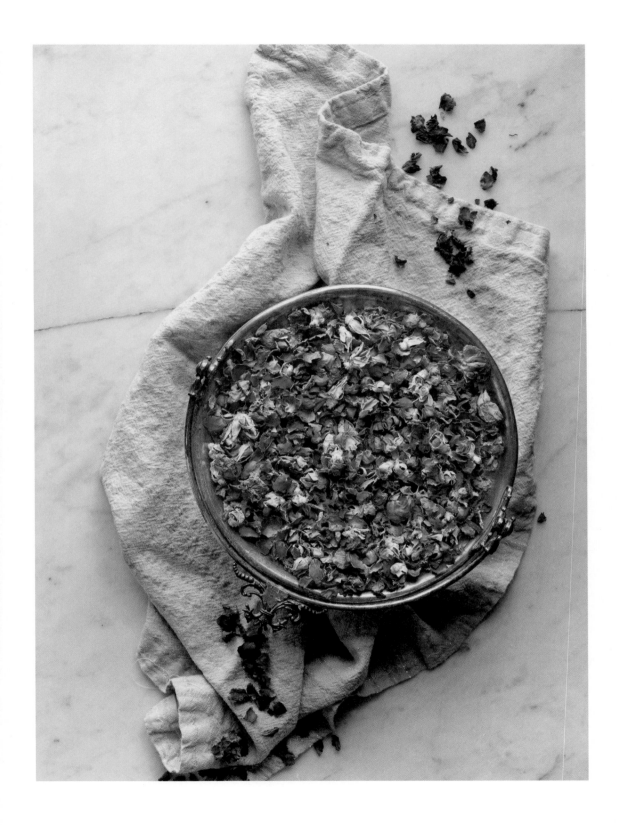

MULTIPURPOSE BODY + MASSAGE OIL

Sweet almond is the carrier oil favoured by aromatherapists for professional massage treatments to the body because it glides across the skin easily and is not absorbed quite as quickly as some of the finer oils, such as light coconut oil or grapeseed oil. The addition of jojoba gives this massage oil a nourishing and replenishing quality and lengthens the shelf life of the blend. The essential oils are chosen to refresh and uplift the senses, and make a good synergy blend of top, middle and base notes for everyday use. This massage oil is suitable for applying to all areas of the body, apart from the face.

Ingredients

- o   50 ml (1¾ fl oz) sweet almond oil
- o   50 ml (1¾ fl oz) jojoba oil
- o   10 drops palmarosa essential oil
- o   10 drops frankincense essential oil
- o   10 drops sweet orange essential oil

Directions

Add the carrier oils to a clean 100-ml (3½-fl oz) tinted glass bottle with a pump lid. Add all the essential oils one by one. Place the pump lid on the bottle and shake well.

To use, warm a little of the oil in your hands before applying it directly to the skin, either for moisturizing or massage.

STRESS-RELIEF BODY + MASSAGE OIL

This is a tried and tested recipe for all types of stress-related conditions which combines several classic healing herbal oils with soothing essential oils. It is suitable for both men and women for feelings of burnout, overwhelm or anxiety, as well as nervous exhaustion. Aromatherapy is especially effective for stress-related issues involving the emotions because essential oils interact with the body, feelings and mind simultaneously.

Ingredients

- o   5 teaspoons St John's wort oil
- o   5 teaspoons calendula oil
- o   5 teaspoons camellia seed oil
- o   5 teaspoons jojoba oil
- o   10 drops sweet marjoram essential oil
- o   10 drops lavender essential oil
- o   10 drops juniper essential oil

Directions

Add all the carrier oils one by one to a clean 100-ml (3½-fl oz) tinted glass bottle with a pump lid. Add the essential oils one by one. Place the pump lid on the bottle and shake well.

To use, warm a little of the oil in your hands before applying it directly to the skin, either for moisturizing or massage.

WOMEN'S BLEND BODY + MASSAGE OIL

Evening primrose oil is traditionally prescribed in herbal medicine for women's complaints, especially hormonal imbalances, the menopause and period pains. Calendula oil is an all-round healing oil for the skin and it is also a tonic for the nervous system. Clary sage oil has a pleasing, sweet, nutty-herbaceous scent, which is especially good for stress and anxiety. Geranium has a balancing and harmonizing effect on the nervous system, while bergamot oil has a soothing effect on the nervous system, although it is reviving and uplifting to the spirit.

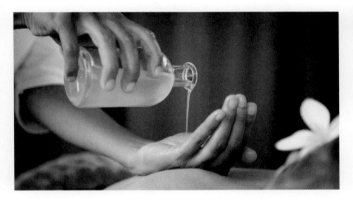

HEALTH TIP

Avoid drinking alcohol when using clary sage essential oil as it has been shown to cause side-effects such as headaches and nausea.

Ingredients

- 60 ml (2 fl oz) grapeseed oil
- 5 teaspoons calendula oil
- 1 tablespoon evening primrose oil
- 10 drops clary sage essential oil
- 10 drops geranium essential oil
- 10 drops bergamot essential oil

Directions

Add all the carrier oils one by one to a clean 100-ml (3½-fl oz) tinted glass bottle with a pump lid. Add the essential oils one by one. Place the pump lid on the bottle and shake well.

To use, warm a little of the oil in your hands before applying it directly to the skin, either for moisturizing or massage. It is best applied after a bath or shower when the skin is warm, or a little can be rubbed gently into the abdomen in a clockwise direction for period pains.

MEN'S BLEND AROMATIC BODY + MASSAGE OIL

Grapeseed oil a rich source of linoleic acid (omega 6) which is important for protecting skin cell membranes and conditioning the skin. Avocado oil is very rich in nutrients, including vitamins A, D, B1, B2 pantothenic acid, E, lecithin and essential fatty acids. Wheatgerm includes vitamin E, which helps improve skin elasticity, while nourishing and moisturizing skin cells. Adding 5 per cent of wheatgerm oil to a body oil also acts as natural preservative lengthening the life of the blend, plus adding valuable nutrients. The woody aromatic oils together with myrrh oil create an effective synergy which is both healing and restorative for the senses.

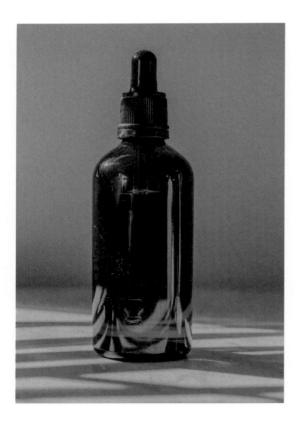

Ingredients

- 60 ml (2 fl oz) grapeseed oil
- 2 tablespoons calendula oil
- 1 teaspoon avocado oil
- 1 teaspoon wheatgerm oil (or vitamin E oil)
- 10 drops cypress essential oil
- 10 drops sandalwood essential oil
- 10 drops myrrh essential oil

Directions

Add all the carrier oils one by one to a clean 100-ml (3½-fl oz) tinted glass bottle with a pump lid. Add all the essential oils one by one. Place the pump lid on the bottle and shake.

To use, warm a little of the oil in your hands before applying it directly to the skin, either for moisturizing or massage.

CHILDREN'S GENTLE BODY + MASSAGE OIL

Children love to be massaged! It is both comforting and relaxing for all ages – but we need to be aware that a child's skin is very delicate and their body much smaller (depending on their age), so the proportion of essential oils in any recipe needs to be reduced substantially. All the active ingredients also need to be very gentle on the skin – peach kernel, calendula, chamomile, lavender and mandarin are all suitable for children being very safe, mild oils. See also the Safety Guidelines on page 168.

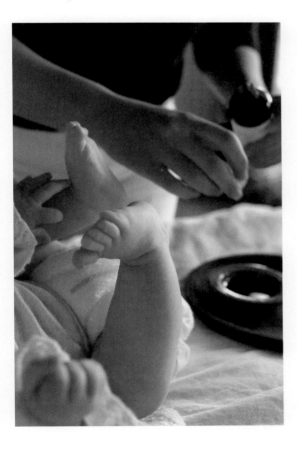

Ingredients

o   80 ml (2¾ f l oz) peach kernel oil
o   4 teaspoons calendula oil
o   6 drops chamomile essential oil
o   6 drops lavender essential oil
o   6 drops mandarin essential oil

Directions

Add all the carrier oils one by one to a clean 100-ml (3½-fl oz) tinted glass bottle with a pump lid. Add all the essential oils one by one. Place the pump lid on the bottle and shake.

To use, warm a little of the oil in your hands before applying it directly to the skin, either for moisturizing or massage.

ORANGE, ROSE + BENZOIN MASSAGE MELTS

These delicious aromatic melts, based on creamy butters and nourishing herbal and aromatic oils, are great to make as a batch for future enjoyment. If you like, you can also try out different blends within one batch. These scented treats are fun to make with children and make lovely gifts. They can then be used either for self-massage or for massaging another person, as they melt readily into the skin. They are best applied after bathing or showering to hydrate, scent and nourish the skin.

Ingredients

- 1 silicon tray with 6 x 15-ml (1-fl oz) moulds
- 4 teaspoons cocoa butter
- 4 teaspoons shea butter
- 2 tablespoons St John's wort oil
- 2 tablespoons calendula oil
- 5 drops rose essential oil
- 5 drops benzoin essential oil
- 2 drops orange essential oil
- Dried rose or calendula petals for decoration (optional)

Directions

Place a glass jug or bowl over a small saucepan of water to create a bain-marie or use a double boiler. Bring the water to the boil, and then reduce to a simmer.

Add the shea and cocoa butter and the herb-infused oils. Keep on the heat until everything has melted, then remove from the heat and stir well as the mixture cools. Add the essential oils to the bowl and mix well.

Measure about 1 tablespoon of the mix into each mould, depending on the size. Press dried flowers on the top of each one, if using, and leave to cool.

Remove when fully set – check after 1 hour. This will depend on the size of the mould or the number of cases you have used.

To use, massage the melt into the body using warm hands. Store the melts in a cotton bag or wrap individually in brown paper tied with string.

VARIATION

For very pretty decorative melts, ideal for gifting, use individual cupcake cases or flower-shaped silicon moulds instead of square moulds.

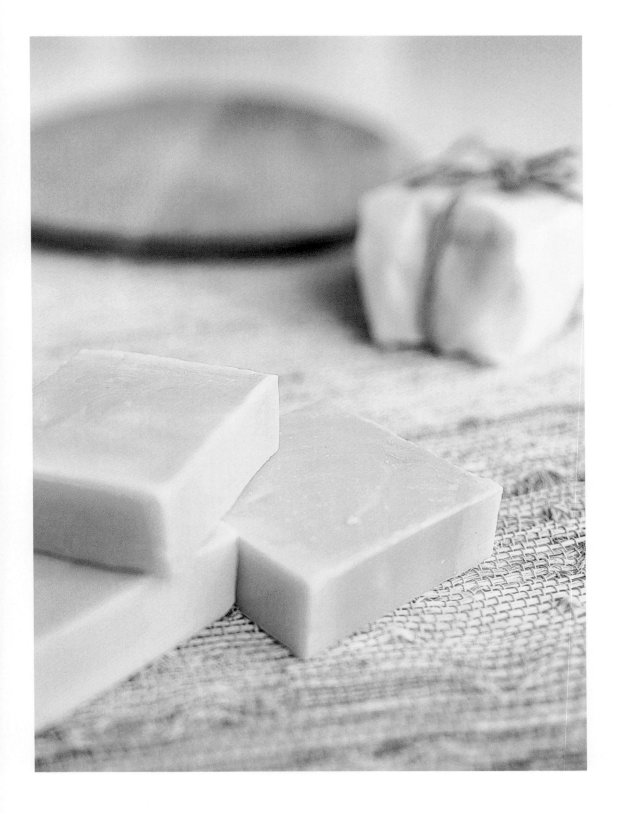

REFRESHING LEG + FOOT MIST

This is a cooling, refreshing panacea for tired legs and feet – it also has a soothing and deodorizing effect. Spearmint acts as a light antiperspirant and tea tree water has outstanding bactericidal, antiseptic and antifungal properties, making it useful for trips at home or abroad. All the essentials included here have excellent antiseptic and anti-inflammatory properties, which make this aqua spritz your go-to natural travel companion.

Ingredients

- 2 teaspoons witch hazel water
- 1 teaspoon vegetable glycerine
- 1 teaspoon aloe vera water or gel
- 8 drops white thyme essential oil
- 8 drops lavender essential oil
- 8 drops peppermint essential oil
- 8 drops rosemary essential oil
- 40 ml (1½ fl oz) tea tree water
- 40 ml (1½ fl oz) spearmint water

Directions

Add the witch hazel, vegetable glycerine and aloe vera or gel one by one to a clean 100-ml (3½-fl oz) tinted glass bottle with an atomizer lid. Add the essential oils, then the tea tree and spearmint waters. Place the atomizer lid on and give the bottle a good shake.

To use, spray liberally onto tired legs and feet.

For optimum refreshment on the skin, keep your foot mist cool in the fridge – don't forget to label it!

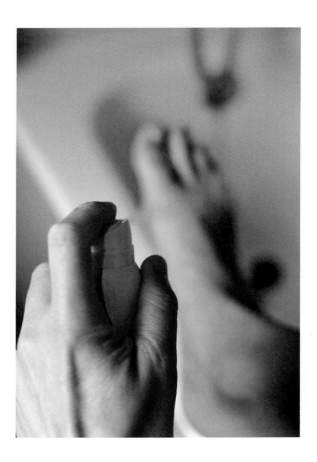

BACTERICIDAL FOOT BALM

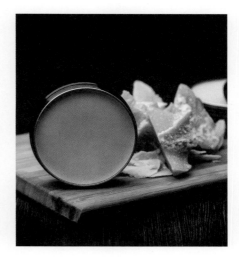

This powerful antiseptic blend is ideal for protecting the feet from all kinds of fungal and bactericidal infections that can affect nails, as well as acting as a healing balm. Infections can be picked up in public swimming pools, for example, but feet also suffer from being trapped in shoes or boots over the winter months especially. Liberate your feet and let them breathe – walk barefoot whenever possible as this stimulates the organs within the body and acts as a kind of natural massage too.

Ingredients

- 1 tablespoon beeswax
- 1½ tablespoons cocoa butter
- 2 teaspoons shea butter
- 2 tablespoons light coconut oil
- 2 teaspoons calendula oil
- 1 teaspoon wheatgerm oil
- 3 drops sweet marjoram essential oil
- 3 drops lemongrass essential oil
- 3 drops tea tree essential oil
- 3 drops peppermint essential oil

Directions

Place a glass jug or bowl over a small saucepan of water to create a bain-marie or use a double boiler. Bring the water to the boil and then reduce to a simmer. Add the beeswax, butters and coconut, calendula and wheatgerm oils to the bowl. Keep on the heat until everything has melted, stirring regularly.

Once the mixture is melted, remove from the heat, add the essential oils one by one and stir well.

Pour the balm mix into a glass jar or aluminium tin to store and allow to set.

Once the balm has set, it is ready to use and enjoy. Massage gently into dry or damp feet (after a foot bath) once a day or as required, paying attention to the soles of your feet and toe nails. Best used within 6 months.

GARDENER'S RESTORATIVE HAND SALVE

Gardening can be tough on the hands – I know because I am a passionate gardener. The hands are constantly exposed to the effects of the sun and chilling weather – quite apart from all the scrapes and scratches that inevitably occur when working in the garden. This is a restorative blend using rich nourishing butters, healing oils, plus aromatic oils, all with good regenerative qualities. Don't forget to apply sun protection on your hands before you go out!

Ingredients

- 60 grams (2 oz) shea butter
- 2 tablespoons aloe vera butter
- 2 tablespoons avocado oil
- 2 teaspoons wheatgerm oil
- 2 teaspoons borage oil
- 4 drops sweet basil essential oil
- 4 drops palmarosa essential oil
- 4 drops rose geranium essential oil

Directions

Place a glass jug or bowl over a small saucepan of water to create a bain-marie or use a double boiler. Bring the water to the boil and then reduce to a simmer. Add the butters and the avocado, wheatgerm and borage oils. Keep on the heat until everything has melted, stirring regularly.

Once the mixture is ready, remove from the heat, add the essential oils one by one and stir well.

Pour the balm mix into a glass jar or aluminium tin to store and allow the balm to set.

Once it has set, it is ready to use and enjoy. To use, apply to hands and nails, ideally after using a hand or body scrub. Best used within 6 months.

HEALTH TIP

Shea butter makes a wonderful medicinal ointment for the relief of itching due to dermatitis, eczema or psoriasis, and it soothes sunburn too.

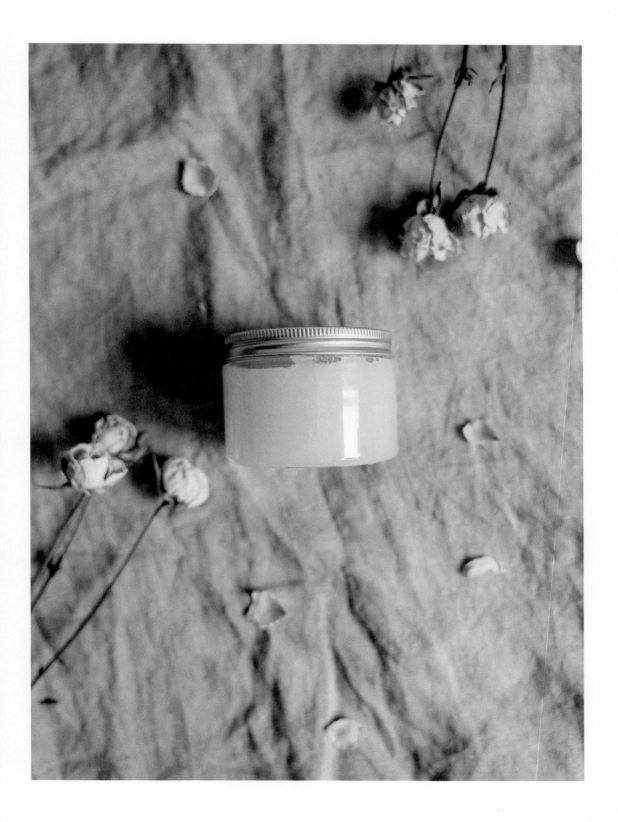

NOURISHING CUTICLE + NAIL OIL

This deeply moisturizing oil can be applied to both fingernails and toenails. It is best applied once your nails have softened after taking a warm bath or shower. Try to use it daily – keep it on your bedside table or next to your bathroom sink so it is easy to remember to give your nails some TLC every day.

Ingredients

- 1 teaspoon avocado oil
- 1 teaspoon light coconut oil
- ¼ teaspoon vitamin E oil
- 2 drops rose geranium essential oil
- 2 drops tea tree essential oil
- 2 drops myrrh essential oil

Directions

Add the avocado, coconut and vitamin E oils to a 10-ml (⅓-fl oz) tinted glass bottle with a pipette top and add in the essential oils. Place the pipette top on and shake well to combine.

Use 1–2 pipettes per hand and foot each day. Massage well into the nail beds and cuticles then leave the oils to soak in, ideally overnight.

EVERYDAY NOURISHING BEARD OIL

This multipurpose beard oil to impart shine and health to the beard, is based on a trinity of super-nourishing and conditioning botanical oils. The aromatic essential oil blend gives it a pleasing woody-green, slightly exotic fragrance.

Ingredients

- 4 teaspoons jojoba oil
- 1 teaspoon argan oil
- 1 teaspoon avocado oil (refined)
- 3 drops bay essential oil
- 3 drops cedarwood essential oil
- 2 drops rosemary essential oil
- 1 drop patchouli essential oil

Directions

Add the jojoba, argan and avocado oils to a clean 30-ml (1-fl oz) tinted glass bottle with a pipette top. Next, add the essential oils one by one. Screw on the pipette top and shake.

To use, apply 1–2 pipettes to a clean dry or damp face to maintain a healthy beard, ideally daily.

LIFESTYLE TIP

The cuticle and beard oil make great presents as a 'his and hers' gift set.

CONDITIONING HOT OIL TREATMENT FOR ALL HAIR TYPES

A homemade hot oil treatment helps nourish the hair with vitamins and minerals. Always apply a hair oil conditioner to dry hair, not wet hair, and follow by shampooing and rinsing with water. If your hair is already wet, the oil in this natural hair conditioning recipe will sit on top of the water and not penetrate your hair and scalp.

Oil, by nature, is very hydrating, so consider the texture and consistency of your hair and then follow the recipe best suited to your hair type. If you tend to have a greasy scalp but dry, split, damaged ends, only apply the conditioning oil to the ends of your hair. If your hair is coarse, thick and dry, oil treatments can be enjoyed more regularly and applied to the full length of your hair.

VARIATION

For a quick and simple hot oil treatment, simply heat 1–3 tablespoons of vegetable oil on the hob or in a microwave for 60 seconds, then add 3–6 drops of essential oil.

Ingredients

Oily hair

- 1–3 tablespoons jojoba oil
- 1 drop cedarwood essential oil
- 1 drop clary sage essential oil
- 1 drop rosemary essential oil

Normal hair

- 1–3 tablespoons argan oil
- 1 drop lavender essential oil
- 1 drop chamomile essential oil
- 1 drop rosemary essential oil

Damaged / dyed hair (or as an after-sun treatment)

- 1½ tablespoons avocado oil
- 1½ tablespoons castor oil
- 1 drop chamomile essential oil
- 1 drop lavender essential oil
- 1 drop bay essential oil

Directions

Place a glass jug or bowl over a small saucepan of water to create a bain-marie or use a double boiler. Bring the water to the boil and then reduce to a simmer. Add the vegetable base oils and allow the oil to heat to a temperature that is bearable on the skin (not too hot!).

Once warmed, add the essential oils and apply to dry hair immediately using your hands or a comb.

Once the hair is covered with the oil, wrap your head in a towel or shower cap and leave on for at least 20 minutes.

Apply shampoo all over the hair before rinsing off with water; this will remove the oil effectively and leave your hair shiny rather than greasy.

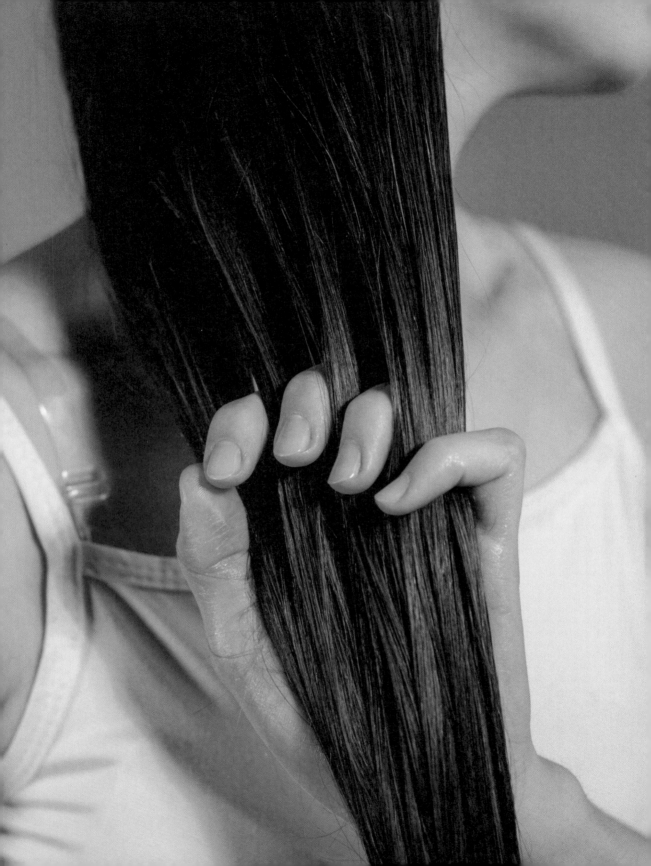

SCALP MASSAGE BOOST FOR SHINY HAIR

Hair health starts with the scalp, and the best remedy for treating a dry scalp, as well as dandruff, is an oil treatment massage. Massaging the head and scalp with natural oils improves the circulation, encourages hair growth and reduces dry skin and dandruff. Using your fingertips, rub about a tablespoon of this warm conditioning blend into your hair and massage well into the scalp, working into the roots to soften and loosen dry skin. Suitable for all hair types, but especially for promoting hair growth and health. Try using this conditioning blend once a week.

Ingredients

- 50 ml (1¾ fl oz) of jojoba oil
- 2 tablespoons argan oil
- 4 teaspoons coconut oil
- 35 drops rosemary essential oil
- 20 drops lavender essential oil
- 15 drops tea tree essential oil

Directions

Pour the jojoba, argan and coconut oils in a clean 100-ml (3½-fl oz) tinted glass bottle with a pump top. Add the essential oils one by one. Put on the lid and shake thoroughly to ensure all the ingredients are well combined.

To use, warm a small amount of the oil in your palms, then massage your head by placing your fingertips on the scalp and gently rubbing the oil into the skin in small circles for about 5 to 10 minutes.

Cover with a shower cap or aluminium foil, followed by a warm, damp towel, and leave on for 15 minutes to 1 hour. Finish by shampooing, conditioning and then rinsing well. If your scalp is very dry, massage with oil before every shampoo.

MOROCCAN CLAY HAIR MASK

Mud and clay are great for oily or flaky scalps, as they help to tackle excess oil and grease and remove toxins. Massaging a mud-based mask into the scalp once a week will help to eliminate grease, which can make the hair look lifeless and flat. Rhassoul clay and rosemary water give the hair body and shine. The aromatic oils all have antiseptic properties, which will eliminate scalp problems, including dandruff. If you have greasy hair, avoid very hot water while washing or rinsing as this stimulates the sebaceous glands.

Ingredients

- 50 grams (1¾ oz) rhassoul clay
- 50 ml (1¾ fl oz) rosemary flower water
- 1 drop tea tree essential oil
- 1 drop peppermint essential oil
- 1 drop rosemary essential oil

Directions

Put the clay into a bowl, and slowly stir in the rosemary water to create a paste. Add the essential oils and stir.

For oily hair, massage the mask onto dry hair and leave for up to 20 minutes. To wash off, apply shampoo directly onto dry hair, then rinse and repeat several times to ensure the oiliness is gone. For normal or dry hair, massage onto wet hair before shampooing and conditioning.

HERBAL RINSE WITH APPLE CIDER VINEGAR

This a traditional home hair rinse recipe based on apple cider vinegar – preferably with the 'mother' – plus rosemary and herb infusions. Applying apple cider vinegar to your haircare routine regularly will help keep your scalp healthy by warding off bacteria and balancing the pH levels and will also stimulate hair growth.

Ingredients

- 6 sprigs fresh or dried rosemary
- 12 fresh or dried sage leaves
- ½–1 cup apple cider vinegar
- Spring water

Directions

Fill a sterilized glass jar with the herbs, trimming them to size if necessary. Cover the herbs with apple cider vinegar and leave in a dark place for roughly 4 weeks, shaking the jar every few days.

Strain out the herbs, then seal the jar and store the vinegar somewhere cool and dry.

To apply the hair rinse, use equal parts herb vinegar and water: for example, 2 tablespoons of vinegar with 2 tablespoons of water. Massage the herbal rinse into wet hair and scalp after shampooing.

ROSEMARY + WHITE CLAY DRY SHAMPOO

A useful dry shampoo to get rid of any greasy build-up between washes, this uses kaolin (or lavender powder), which is very lightweight in texture. A few drops of rosemary essential oil gives it a delightful scent and adds shine to the hair. Remember to remove any clay residue after applying by brushing through the hair thoroughly.

Ingredients

- 10 drops rosemary essential oil
- 2 tablespoons kaolin / white clay (or lavender powder)

Directions

Add the ingredients to a clean 30-ml (1-fl oz) tinted glass bottle with a pump top. Put on the lid and shake thoroughly to ensure the ingredients are well combined.

Put a small amount into your hands and massage through your hair and onto your scalp, rubbing in small circles with your fingertips for a couple of minutes. Brush through to remove any powdery residue.

SOAPWORT + SEA MOSS SHAMPOO

Although this dry herbal mixture doesn't foam like most shampoos, it does provide a natural botanical alternative to liquid shampoos and leaves the hair smelling fresh. It is best to make a fresh batch for each wash, using the amounts below.

Ingredients

- 50 grams (1¾ oz) soapwort root
- 2 tablespoons Irish sea moss
- 2 tablespoons dried herbs — any mixture of chamomile, nettle, rosemary and peppermint
- 2 drops rosemary or peppermint essential oil

Directions

Add the dry ingredients to a large glass beaker or jug and pour in 300 ml (10½ fl oz) of boiling water. Leave to cool, stirring occasionally, for a few minutes.

Strain the herbs and, being quite vigorous with this process, use a spoon or rolling pin to push the liquid through a sieve. You should now be left with a jelly-like shampoo substance. Add the essential oils.

To apply, massage into your scalp and hair as you would a regular shampoo, then rinse.

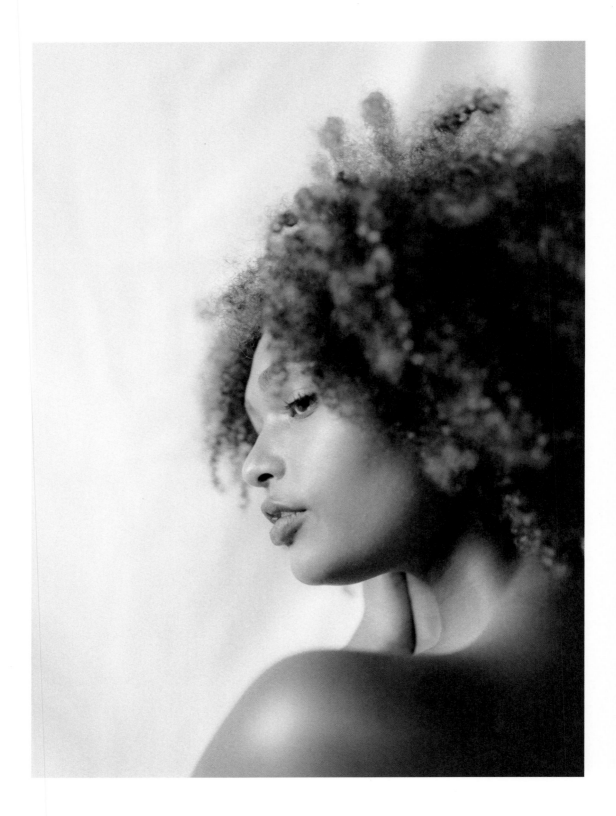

'Your health begins with your cells, because everything about you begins with your cells ... and the quality of your hair and your nails and your skin.'

CAMERON DIAZ, *THE LONGEVITY BOOK*

3 + SKINCARE

A Personalized Skincare Approach

In aromatherapy, essential oils are utilized for their versatile therapeutic properties and outstanding skincare applications. Oils such as rose, neroli, lavender, frankincense and myrrh all have potent antioxidant properties, which prevents the decomposition of organic cells and thus inhibits the ageing process. Modern scientific tests have proven that essential oils can stimulate cellular generation and rejuvenate the dermal tissue, thus keeping the skin looking radiant from within. Since essential oils are absorbed readily through our skin, penetrating deep into the dermal layers, they provide the ideal active ingredients for creating remarkable skincare products, body treatments and other healthcare formulations.

Maintaining healthy, youthful-looking skin depends on everyday skincare as well as on general health. Beware of products containing mineral oil as they are not absorbed into the lower dermal layers where the newly emerging cells require optimum nourishment. Most commercial toners also contain alcohol, which actually has a drying effect on the skin and may cause irritation and dryness, as can other synthetic ingredients found in many creams and lotions. In contrast, natural vegetable oils, combined with selected essential oils are ideal cosmetic aids because they are highly penetrative and can reach the small blood capillaries in the deeper dermal layers, thus rejuvenating the skin from within. Likewise, gentle, alcohol-free flower waters tone and refresh without dehydrating the skin and have a mild bactericidal action alongside. Essential oils and other botanical oils can also be very effective in treating and rejuvenating damaged skin, caused by excessive sun exposure or other factors, such as scars or stretch marks.

Our skin is made up of three layers: the surface layer is called the epidermis, which acts as a primary barrier; the middle layer called the dermis, contains blood vessels, nerve endings, hair roots and sweat glands; while the deeper subcutaneous fat layer contains the larger blood vessels and nerves. The top layer of the skin or epidermis also plays a key role in retaining moisture due to a unique mixture of amino acids and salts found in these cells. If we use strong soaps or detergents, however, these valuable components are washed away and our skin loses some of its ability to retain water. The middle and deeper cellular layers are more concerned with nourishing the skin and regulating moisture levels.

Water is the way nutrients are carried to the tissues of our skin and is essential to keep these deeper dermal layers moisturized, thus maintaining their elasticity. But apart from keeping our skin hydrated and clean by bathing, and since the skin is our primary barrier against pathogens, it is also very important to apply water to our skin via creams and water-based lotions, as this will make a visible difference to its overall health. Water plumps up the skin from within, giving it a vital and glowing appearance, making it less wrinkled and helping to delay the signs of ageing, as well as flushing out any impurities and keeping the outer dermal layer free of spots.

One of the pioneers of aromatherapy, the French cosmetologist Marguerite Maury, considered that essential oils were especially valuable as skincare agents to promote a youthful complexion and prevent the signs of ageing. In her groundbreaking book *The Secret of Life and Youth*, she outlined how essential oils can

be used to rejuvenate and renew the skin by cleansing, revitalizing and nourishing the cellular tissues at their deepest dermal layers. She also advocated that radiant beauty and longevity could be optimized via an 'individual prescription' or IP, a personalized skincare regime and bespoke formulations based on each person's unique requirements. As a biochemist specializing in research on essential oils, my mother Kerttu Ajanko was also well versed in the remarkable and unique biochemical make-up of aromatic oils and recommended their use for personalized skincare treatments long before the term 'aromatherapy' became fashionable.

The unique value of being able to create your own skincare products at home is they can be tailored not only to your skin type and to your unique personality but also to your fragrance preferences. Creating a personalized facial serum, for example, is a valuable way to experiment with making an 'individual prescription', which can then be used as part of your everyday routine. Facial oils are made up in much the same way as body oils, except that the carrier oils and essential oils are more finely adapted to your skin type. Suitable base carrier oils include sweet almond, light coconut, grapeseed, jojoba, rosehip seed, apricot kernel or argan – additional highly nutritious or 'booster' oils such as avocado, wheatgerm, borage or evening primrose can also be added to the blend to enhance the properties of the blend for specific types of skin. Some people are nervous

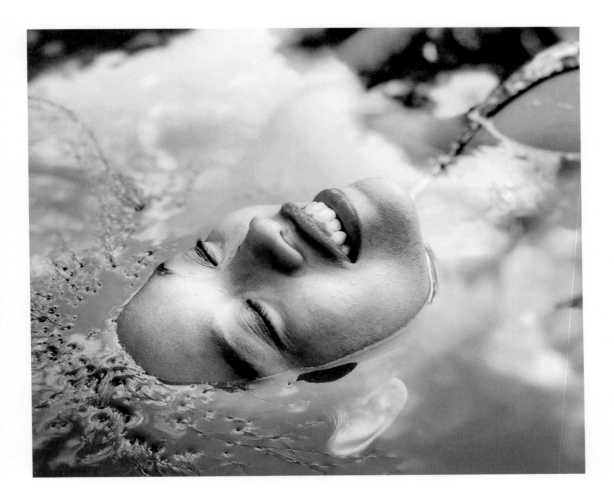

of applying oil to the face, especially to oily or blemish-prone skin, but the results will speak for themselves! Apart from nourishing and hydrating the skin, facial oils can also help overcome skin complaints such as acne or scarring.

It is best to apply a facial oil before bed, as night-time is the period when our skin can absorb nutrients most readily, away from the adverse effects of the sun, central heating, pollutants or make-up. It is important to always keep concentrated essential oils well away from the eyes.

Within a wider therapeutic context, aromatherapy is very helpful for both physical and emotional complaints, the two being intimately connected. Essential oils are unique therapeutic agents, in that they not only exert their effects on a physiological level when they are applied to the skin or inhaled into the lungs, but they also exert a psychological and emotional effect via our sense of smell and the limbic system when we breathe in their volatile vapours. Many common skin complaints, such as eczema, acne or rosacea, are exacerbated by conditions like anxiety or depression, and tend to flare up during times of stress. Heat rash and hives can also be exacerbated or brought on by stress – even the condition of our hair is affected by our emotional state. In this case, an aromatherapy style of holistic approach to problematic skin complaints can be very valuable.

Many other ingredients also play a part in the art of aromatic formulation in the context of skincare, such as different types of clay, flower waters, botanical herbs and carrier oils. Today, the wisdom of using individually tailored skincare products, which are perfectly suited to the needs of each individual, is gaining ever-increasing popularity. The art of creating our own individual skin and beauty treatments, such as aromatic creams, clay masks, facial serums and oils at home, while individualizing them to our own personal needs, makes perfect sense for a whole range of reasons, not least because we can create skincare formulations that are ideally suited to our particular skin type, but we can also save money by using high-quality ingredients rather than off-the-shelf items and be more eco-friendly by cutting out superfluous packaging.

Creating a tailored individual skincare routine may also need to be adjusted depending on the time of year and our immediate environment. During the spring and summer our skin is often exposed to the damaging effects from ultraviolet rays, yet this damage is not fully apparent until afterwards – perhaps even 10 to 20 years later!

That is why it is so important to protect our skin during the summer months, especially when we are young, to help avoid the signs of ageing occurring prematurely in the future. It is important to always wear a suitable SPF sunscreen on areas of our skin which are exposed to the sun. It is good to be aware that this is different to a sunblock, which would also block the absorption of vitamin D from the sun's rays. Nevertheless, we can still help to overcome existing problems such as wrinkles, blotches or dark spots – or at least minimize the damage – by applying so called 'booster' oils to our skin in a targeted manner. By this I mean applying concentrated antioxidant oils locally, which encourages cellular regeneration, such as so-called 'carrot' oil – made from the sea algae *Dunaliella salina* which is very high in carotene – as well as borage oil, pressed from the seeds of the beautiful starflower, due to its high gamma-linolenic acid content.

Ultraviolet rays cause collagen to break down in our skin which is vital for maintaining elasticity and tone. But by increasing our daily intake of vitamin C, both via our diet and through the topical application of oils high in vitamins, we can help to rebuild this collagen naturally. Aromatic flower waters also are beneficial when applied directly to the face and body during the summer months to help keep the skin hydrated. In contrast, during autumn and winter, due to the colder temperatures and increased exposure to central heating, our skin can start to look pale and dull. It therefore makes sense to feed our skin on a daily basis using super-nourishing oils to ensure our complexion stays hydrated and radiates a healthy, fresh glow. This means using facial oils rather than water-based lotions on our face, neck and hands and including rich oils in our daily skincare routine, as well as applying conditioning oils to our body, hair and nails. Taking a liquid vitamin D supplement as an alternative to the vitamin D obtained from sunshine is also valuable during the colder months.

Many people typically have a skin type which is close to normal, but society – particularly the cosmetic industry – has conditioned us to believe that our complexion is constantly a problem which we somehow need to fix. In this way, confidence in our appearance remains forever out of reach since we're always trying to achieve a look that we currently don't have. Natural beauty is about enjoying the skin we are in, and simply augmenting our unique features. It is good to remember that growing old is also an entirely natural process and has its own type of beauty when we age gracefully. When we examine our own skin, we may find that we don't necessarily fit into one category – such as dry, sensitive or oily – this is because our skin can change according to various factors including our environment, the food we eat, as well as our age. Different skin types require individual treatment, but the truth is that most of us have some form of combination skin – or a skin that is ever changing like the seasons! In fact,

people often have different skin types in specific areas of their face.

The three main skin problems which need to be addressed are spots and blemishes, people with very sensitive complexions and those with very dry skin. Individuals often develop blemished skin, particularly teenagers or those who live in cities, as a reaction to hormonal changes or to environmental pollution, in which case this can be remedied using natural treatments. Those with very delicate or sensitive skin, who can be prone to thread veins, need to be careful when they apply any products to their skin to avoid sensitization issues. Mature skin is another type of skin that needs proper care and protection, especially if the skin is very dry. You should therefore adapt your daily skincare routine to your individual needs as well as to your environment. It is also beneficial to treat yourself to a special 'home spa' treatment session once a week, to include personalized masks, scrubs and conditioners.

In the skincare recipe section, you will find formulations for each skin type, including dry, oily and mature complexions, as well as ways to treat other conditions, such as blemishes, cracked lips or sunburned skin. These recipes provide a general guideline for each skin type, but since we often have different areas on our faces – for example, an oily T-zone but dry and delicate areas around the eyes – these factors also need to be taken into account when applying your personalized skincare routine.

SKINCARE RECIPES

The most basic three-step skincare routine to be repeated twice daily consists of cleansing, toning and moisturizing. This routine should be carried out both in the morning and evening using personalized formulations. Other skincare products, such as eye serums, scrubs and masks, can be applied as required, perhaps once a week. A general tip is to always to start with the lightest-weight product first then end with the heaviest consistency – cleansing lotions, toning waters, facial oils, serums and finally any thicker moisturizing creams or balms. Many of the proportions used in the recipes here, such as the face masks, are for single use only, whereas the facial oils can last several months. The cleansing recipes include essential oils as optional only. Don't forget to label your natural skincare products especially if you put them in the fridge! Note: all essential oils should be kept well away from the eyes – rinse with water immediately if contact should occur.

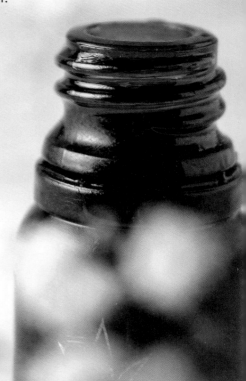

QUICK COCONUT CLEANSER FOR ALL SKIN TYPES

It is important to cleanse your face daily to maintain a clear complexion. No other part of your body is exposed to as many chemicals – from make-up, air pollution or just from the dust or grime in the air. Gradually, a build-up of dirt and grease seeps into the pores of the skin, clogging them up. Eventually, the skin pores can develop keratin caps that keep the sebum trapped in the follicles. Light coconut oil is a gentle yet thorough cleanser as the fine, dispersing texture of the oil enables it to seep deep into the pores and hair follicles, dissolving any hardened sebum. Applying a steaming cloth to the face further gently exfoliates the skin, helping to remove any dirt, impurities or dead skin cells from deep within, leaving the surface dermal layers renewed and hydrated. This can also be used on the eye area to remove make-up.

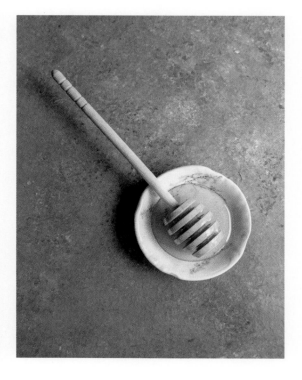

Ingredients

○   ½ tablespoon light coconut oil
○   1 teaspoon raw honey (optional)

Directions

Combine the coconut oil and honey, if using, in your hand or a small jar, then massage it into your skin gently, using gentle upward strokes to remove any dirt. This same routine can also be applied at night to remove make-up.

Saturate a flannel or muslin cloth under a semi-hot tap or under a shower, then wring it out and place the warm flannel onto your face, leaving it for 1 to 2 minutes.

Gently rub the mixture off your face using the flannel or cloth, until the skin no longer feels greasy.

REPLENISHING CLEANSING BALM FOR DRY OR MATURE SKIN

For dry, delicate or mature skin, jojoba oil has an extra moisturizing effect so is preferable to light coconut, or you could include both oils in a 50:50 ratio. Jojoba oil has a remarkable biochemical likeness to the sebum in our skin, so it also makes an excellent cleanser by lifting dirt out from deep within the pores. A single drop of sea buckthorn oil contains 190 different bioactive compounds and imparts a lovely bright orange tint to the balm too. This balm leaves your skin clean, supple and soft after cleansing.

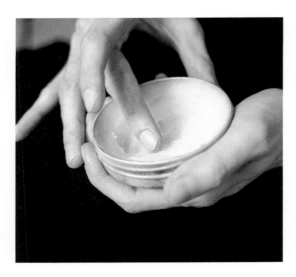

Ingredients

○ 1 tablespoon beeswax
○ 90 ml (3 fl oz) jojoba oil
○ 2 tablespoons sea buckthorn oil
○ 1 tablespoon aloe vera butter
○ 6 drops neroli 5 per cent essential oil
○ 6 drops sandalwood 5 per cent essential oil

Directions

Place a glass jug or bowl over a small saucepan of water to create a bain-marie or use a double boiler. Bring the water to the boil and then reduce to a simmer. Add the beeswax, jojoba oil, sea buckthorn oil and aloe vera butter and stir with a glass rod or wooden spoon until the beeswax melts and it becomes liquid.

Remove from the heat and add the essential oils, stirring vigorously to combine. Decant into a large glass jar or aluminium tin. Leave the product to set for 10 to 20 minutes and place the lid on.

To use, massage onto the face, avoiding the eye area, and remove with a warm cloth.

VARIATION

If you omit the essential oils, this can be used on the eye area to remove make-up, including mascara.

CLAY + HONEY CLEANSER FOR OILY SKIN

CLEANSER FOR COMBINATION/ NORMAL SKIN

Oily and blemished skin can benefit from regular clay and honey cleansing, while normal skin can benefit from it once or twice a week. City dwellers can also use this clay cleanser regularly to remove the daily toxins accumulated from pollution. To make a more detoxifying cleanser, use green clay in this formulation. Alternatively, kaolin is a very gentle clay that is a great choice for dry, dehydrated or sensitive skin. This is best made fresh for each use, but you can also store it in a jar in the fridge and use within a few days if you have any leftover product.

For normal or combination skin, blend the floral water and glycerine with the oils to make a liquid gel and apply to the face, gently massaging in a circular motion. Then saturate a flannel or muslin cloth with semi-hot water and place it on the face for a few minutes before washing off with warm water. This cleanser can also be applied to the skin with cotton wool or bamboo pads before rinsing thoroughly. Store in an atomizer or flip-top lid and use within 6 months.

Ingredients

- 2 tablespoons green or kaolin / white clay
- 2 tablespoons light coconut oil
- 1 tablespoon raw honey
- 1 drop lavender essential oil

Ingredients

- 75 ml (2½ fl oz) geranium flower water (or use fragonia or tea tree water for an oily T-zone)
- 2 tablespoons vegetable glycerine
- 2 tablespoons camellia seed oil
- 2 tablespoons light coconut oil
- 5 drops rosemary essential oil
- 5 drops mandarin essential oil

Directions

Put the clay, oil and honey into a small mixing bowl and stir into a paste using a wooden spoon until well combined.

To use, apply to a dry or damp face with clean hands, using a circular motion. Cover your face for a few minutes with a warm cloth, or, better still, steam your face for 3 to 5 minutes to open up the pores. Rinse the face with warm water.

Directions

Pour the floral waters, glycerine and carrier oils into a clean 100-ml (3½-fl oz) tinted glass bottle. Add the essential oils. Place the lid on and shake well to combine.

To use, apply to a dry or damp face with clean hands or a recyclable cotton pad. Rinse off using warm water.

TONING FACIAL SPRITZ FOR DRY + SENSITIVE SKIN

Natural toners help to restore the skin's protective acid mantle if they are left to dry naturally and are ideally suited for reviving dull or lacklustre skin due to spending too much time indoors exposed to the drying effects of central heating. Most commercial toners use alcohol in their formulations, which is very astringent by nature and dries out the skin further. Dry and sensitive skin benefits from the gentle flower waters of lavender, melissa (lemon balm) and neroli before applying a moisturizer or treatment serum of your choice. In this case, a little vegetable glycerine and aloe vera are added to the formulation for very dry skin.

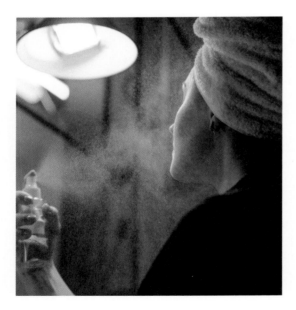

LIFESTYLE TIP

This is a good toning facial spritz for normal skin – it also makes a great travel mist to use when you are on the move, during hot weather or simply as a light perfume.

Ingredients

- 1 teaspoon aloe vera water or gel
- 1 tablespoon vegetable glycerine
- 4 teaspoons melissa water
- 2 tablespoons neroli water
- 2 tablespoons lavender water

Directions

Pour all the ingredients one by one into a clean 100-ml (3½-fl oz) tinted glass bottle using a funnel. Seal the bottle with an atomizer top and shake well. Label the bottle and store in the fridge or in a cool place.

To use, spritz onto the face and neck directly or apply to a recyclable cotton pad and wipe over the face.

3 + Skincare

REHYDRATING MIST FOR COMBINATION/ NORMAL SKIN

Toners are light liquids that are spritzed onto the face and neck directly or applied to a recyclable cotton pad to gently remove the last traces of a cleanser or any remaining makeup before moisturizing. They should always be applied immediately after thoroughly cleansing the skin. Using a gently scented toner is also great way to remove a face mask or face pack leaving your face feeling clean and radiant. However, they can also be used to simply freshen up your face at any time during the day to help rehydrate the skin.

Ingredients

○   1 tablespoon rose water
○   5 teaspoons lavender water
○   5 teaspoons geranium water
○   2 teaspoons vegetable glycerine

Directions

Pour all the ingredients one by one into a clean 100-ml (3½-fl oz) tinted glass bottle with a lid or spray top using a funnel. Seal the lid tightly closed and shake well. Label the bottle and store in the fridge or in a cool place.

To use, spritz onto the face and neck directly or apply to a recyclable cotton pad and wipe over the face.

FRAGONIA TONER FOR OILY SKIN

Flower waters form the basis for making bespoke natural toners that can be particularly good for problem skin. Greasy, blemished and congested skin benefits especially from the application of antiseptic toners containing tea tree water or fragonia water with witch hazel, a tried-and-tested astringent and antioxidant that can help soothe skin inflammation and reduce visible pore size or blackheads. Spearmint water has deodorant effects and is cooling, while rosemary has excellent bactericidal properties. This recipe uses fragonia water, which is milder than tea tree yet very effective.

Ingredients

○   2 teaspoons vegetable glycerine
○   2 tablespoons fragonia water (or tea tree water)
○   2 teaspoons rosemary water
○   2 tablespoons spearmint water
○   2 teaspoons witch hazel

Directions

Add the ingredients one by one to a clean 100-ml (3½-fl oz) tinted glass bottle with an atomizer top. Place the atomizer top on and shake well. Label the bottle and store in the fridge or in a cool place.

To use, spritz onto the face and neck or apply using a recyclable cotton pad.

ROSE + JASMINE TONER FOR MATURE SKIN

Rose and jasmine are both powerful antioxidants, so they are perfect for the care of mature complexions. Mature skin also needs extra moisturizing, so aloe vera gel and glycerine are added to this blend as well as vitamin E. This floral bouquet of aromatic waters has a heavenly scent and will also help to keep your complexion youthful looking and glowing. It is important to always apply a nourishing skin oil or moisturizer to mature skin after toning it on a twice daily basis.

Ingredients

- 5 teaspoons rose water
- 5 teaspoons lavender water
- 5 teaspoons jasmine water
- 1 teaspoons aloe vera water or gel
- 4 teaspoons vegetable glycerine
- 5 drops vitamin E oil

Directions

Pour all the ingredients one by one into a clean 100-ml (3½-fl oz) tinted glass bottle with an atomizer top using a funnel. Add the vitamin E oil. Seal the bottle and shake well to dissolve the vitamin E. Label the bottle and store in a cool place.

To use, spritz onto the face and neck directly or apply using a recyclable cotton pad.

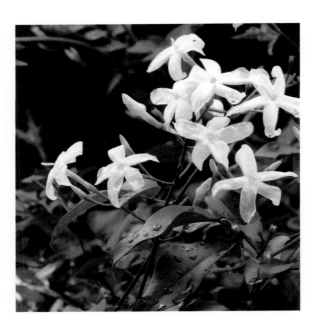

LIFESTYLE TIP

There are many types of recyclable natural cotton pads, organic muslin cloths or flannels (washcloths) available, which are useful for removing makeup and any excess oils or lotions from the skin.

UNSCENTED FACIAL OIL FOR SENSITIVE SKIN

This is a formulation free from essential oils, suitable for all skin types but especially well-matched for sensitive or allergy-prone skin where aromatic oils are best avoided.

These ingredients form a lightweight texture that is readily absorbed into the skin, providing a nourishing treatment for sensitive skin to hydrate, replenish and soothe. Rice bran oil is used extensively in Japan to protect and soothe the skin; Camellia seed oil contains vitamins A, B and E and is rich in minerals while rosehip is an anti-inflammatory with clinically proven results in improving moisture levels in the skin. This oil is suitable for use in the morning and night but is best applied overnight as our skin repairs and regenerates while we sleep.

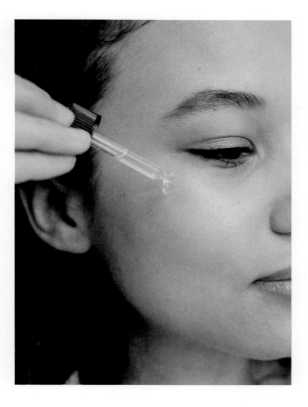

Ingredients

o   1 tablespoon rice bran oil
o   1 teaspoon camellia seed oil
o   1 teaspoon rosehip seed oil
o   1 teaspoon wheatgerm oil
    or vitamin E oil

Directions

Add the carrier oils carefully to a clean 30-ml (1-fl oz) tinted glass bottle with a pipette top. Stir or shake gently to combine all the ingredients. Label the bottle and store in a cool place.

To use, apply to face and neck using upward massage strokes. Ideally, leave on overnight.

FACIAL OIL FOR OILY SKIN

Contrary to widespread belief, an oil formula is one of the best ways to help deal with blemished and oily skin, also working as a long-term preventative treatment. Although it may seem counterintuitive to apply vegetable oils to blemished or greasy skin, as long as you choose the correct base oils – such as jojoba, hazelnut and light coconut oil – all of these oils actually help to rebalance the skin's sebum levels in the deeper dermal layers and therefore help to remove the cause of the problem naturally. This formulation uses gentle fragonia oil, which has a lovely citrus aroma, quite different from tea tree but with many of the same benefits. These ingredients form a balancing blend for oily and blemish-prone skin to protect, purify and hydrate. This oil is suitable for use in the morning and night – but is best applied overnight.

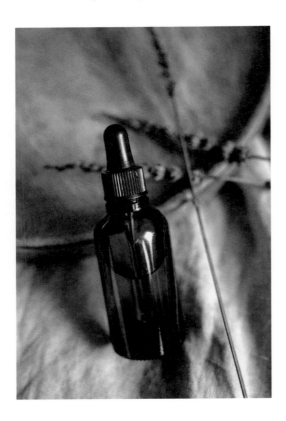

Ingredients

- o 1 tablespoon light coconut oil
- o 1 teaspoon hazelnut oil
- o 2 teaspoons jojoba oil
- o 2 drops sweet myrtle essential oil
- o 2 drops lavender essential oil
- o 2 drops fragonia essential oil

Directions

Add the coconut, hazelnut and jojoba oils carefully to a clean 30-ml (1-fl oz) tinted glass bottle with a pipette top. Add the drops of essential oils one by one. Stir or shake gently to combine all the ingredients.

To use, apply to the face and neck using upward massage strokes. Ideally, leave on overnight.

NOURISHING FACIAL OIL FOR DRY SKIN

Dry skin typically feels tight upon waking and struggles to retain moisture throughout the day. It is also more susceptible to flaking and the appearance of fine lines. Authentic argan oil from Morocco is renowned for providing intense replenishment and hydration to the skin and hair. Macadamia is deeply emollient and a rich source of omegas, while sea buckthorn is an abundant source of many nutrients and minerals. Lavender and mandarin are both gentle essential oils that soothe, heal and promote cell growth. Vetiver essential oil is healing and relaxing to both the skin and psyche.

Together, these ingredients form a nourishing blend for dry skin to comfort, enrich and deeply hydrate.

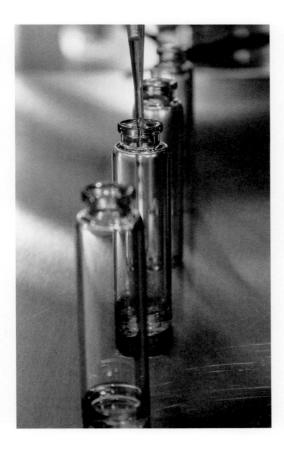

Ingredients

- 2 teaspoons macadamia oil
- 1 teaspoon sea buckthorn oil
- 1 tablespoon argan oil
- 2 drops lavender essential oil
- 2 drops mandarin essential oil
- 2 drops vetiver essential oil

Directions

Add the macadamia, sea buckthorn and argan oils carefully to a clean 30-ml (1-fl oz) tinted glass bottle with a pipette top. Add the drops of essential oils one by one. Stir or shake gently to combine all the ingredients.

To use, apply to face and neck using upward massage strokes morning and night, leaving on overnight if possible.

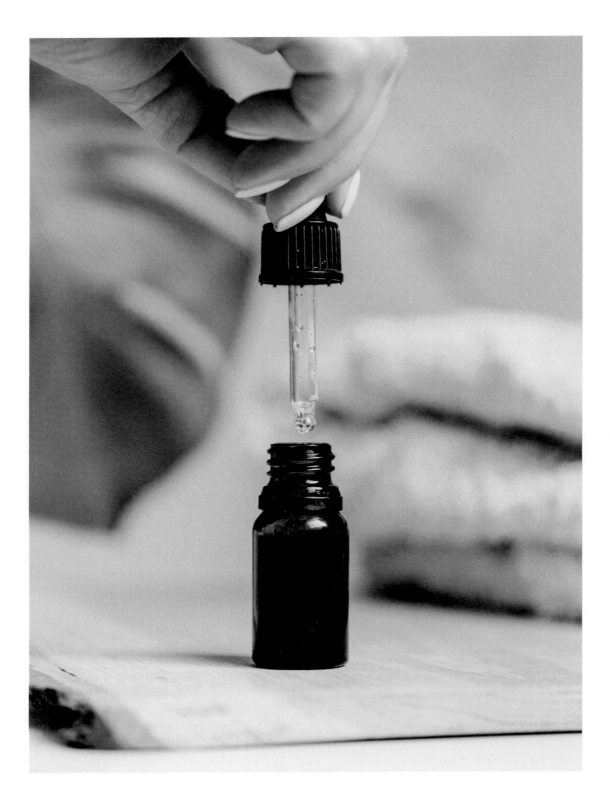

RICH FACIAL OIL FOR MATURE SKIN

As we age, our skin does too, and benefits from extra 'booster' oils, such as borage oil, to help maintain hydration levels, elasticity and suppleness. Also known as starflower, borage is the richest plant source of essential fatty acids including omega 6, making it an optimal choice for mature skin, to restore elasticity and plumpness. It does have a pungent aroma so is best enjoyed in small amounts and combined with other carrier oils. Frankincense is known as the 'king of essential oils' while rose is often called 'queen of the flowers' and together they form a dynamic skin duo with cell-renewing and regenerative properties.

Ingredients

- o   2 teaspoons macadamia oil
- o   1 teaspoon rosehip seed oil
- o   1 teaspoon borage oil
- o   1 teaspoon sea buckthorn oil
- o   1 teaspoon vitamin E oil
- o   2 drops frankincense essential oil
- o   2 drops rose essential oil
- o   2 drops lavender essential oil

Directions

Add the macadamia, rosehip seed, borage, sea buckthorn and vitamin E oils carefully to a clean 30-ml (1-fl oz) tinted glass bottle with a pipette top. Add the drops of essential oils one by one. Stir or shake gently to combine all the ingredients well.

To use, apply to face and neck using upward massage strokes morning and night. Leave on overnight if possible.

HEALTH TIP

Dry skin develops wrinkles much faster than hydrated skin, so it is important to keep mature skin well moisturized using a blended oil or serum suited to your complexion.

REPLENISHING + REJUVENATING ROSE FACE MASK

Rose essential oil is a classic ingredient for mature and sensitive skin: it is also excellent in helping combat troublesome skin complaints such as rosacea, rashes and eczema, especially when these conditions flare up due to stress and anxiety. Rose water has been used for thousands of years to nourish, hydrate and rejuvenate the complexion. This recipe gives a new slant to an age-old formulation: it makes just enough for one mask, so it is best to make a fresh batch each time.

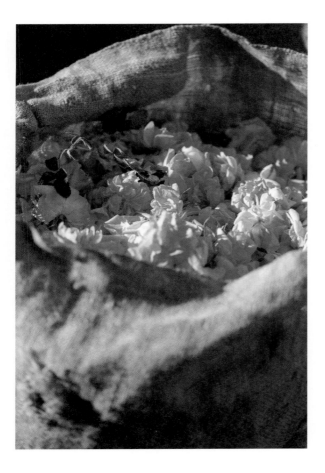

Ingredients

- O 2 teaspoons rosehip powder
- O 1 teaspoon rhassoul clay
- O 3 drops rose essential oil
- O ½ teaspoon rose water, plus extra for finishing

Directions

Add the rosehip powder, clay and rose oil one by one to a bowl, then add the rose water in slowly, stirring with a wooden spoon or glass stirring rod to form a paste.

Use a clean foundation brush or your hands to apply the mixture to the face and neck. Leave on for 10 to 20 minutes, then rinse off with warm water.

Spray the face and use a recyclable cotton pad with the extra rose water to remove the last traces of the mask.

CHARCOAL + FRAGONIA ACNE MASK

This mask or paste is to be applied to spots or to the blemished area only such as the T-zone, not to the entire face. Activated charcoal is one of the best ways of drawing out impurities from the skin while fragonia oil and witch hazel water are antiseptic, bactericidal and healing. Ideally, make a fresh batch for each use.

Ingredients

- o 1 heaped teaspoon activated charcoal
- o 2 drops fragonia essential oil
- o 1 teaspoon raw honey
- o 20 drops witch hazel water, plus extra for finishing

Directions

Add the charcoal, fragonia essential oil and the honey one by one to a bowl, then add the witch hazel water slowly, stirring with a wooden spoon or spatula to form a paste.

To use, apply to acne or the blemished area only. Leave on for 10 to 20 minutes. Rinse with warm water.

Spray the face and use a recyclable cotton pad with the extra witch hazel water to remove any last traces of the acne mask.

SEAWEED + SAGE CLEANSING MASK

French green clay and seaweed are ancient ingredients that have been utilized for centuries around the world for their purifying qualities. Green clay possesses strong absorbent properties that draw out impurities and its antibacterial properties help to ease any irritated skin conditions, while seaweed contains over seventy vitamins and minerals, being particularly rich in iodine. Clary sage oil is balancing and brings stress relief. This mask should be made fresh for each use.

Ingredients

- o 2 teaspoons green clay
- o 1 teaspoon seaweed powder
- o 2 drops clary sage essential oil
- o ½ teaspoon aloe vera water or gel

Directions

Add the clay and seaweed powder to a small bowl, add the clary sage, then add the aloe vera water or gel in slowly, stirring with a spoon or glass rod to form a paste.

Use a clean foundation brush or your hands to apply to the face and neck. Leave on for 10 to 20 minutes. Rinse with warm water. Spray the face and use a recyclable cotton wool pad with your choice of flower water to remove any last traces.

GENTLE PEACH, KAOLIN, OAT + HONEY MASK

This mask is gentle, healing, repairing and good for sunburn and inflamed skin conditions, plus dry and dehydrated skin. It can be enjoyed by young people and children too.

Ingredients

- 2 teaspoons colloidal oatmeal or use a blender or pestle and mortar to grind rolled oats
- 2 teaspoons kaolin / white clay
- 1 teaspoon peach kernel or apricot kernel oil
- 2 teaspoons honey
- 1 teaspoon aloe vera gel or 1 tablespoon Greek yogurt

Directions

If using the rolled oats, grind to a powder in a blender first. Add the oatmeal or oats and the kaolin in a small bowl. Add the peach kernel oil (or apricot kernel) and honey slowly, stirring to make a paste. Then add the aloe vera gel (or yogurt), stirring with a wooden spoon or glass rod to form a paste.

Use a clean foundation brush or your hands to apply to the face and neck. Leave on for 10 to 20 minutes. Rinse with warm water and a cloth or muslin. Use a recyclable cotton wool pad with a gentle flower water to remove the last traces.

PURIFYING FACIAL SCRUB

Regular exfoliation can remove debris, dirt and dead skin cells, thus making the skin appear more refined and even in texture. Kaolin or white clay is the gentlest and mildest of all the clays available, making it suitable for regular use. Rice bran provides a gentle exfoliation and aids the skin in balancing moisture by removing excess oils. Palmarosa oil has an uplifting scent and balances the sebum production in the skin to help maintain oil levels, along with beneficial bactericidal properties. This mask should be made fresh for each use and can be used once a week as part of your skincare routine.

Ingredients

- 1 teaspoon apricot kernel oil
- 2 teaspoons kaolin / white clay
- 1 teaspoon rice bran or rice bran powder
- ½ teaspoon Dead Sea salt
- 2 drops palmarosa essential oil

Directions

Add the apricot kernel oil, kaolin clay, rice bran and Dead Sea salt one by one to a bowl, then add the palmarosa essential oil and mix well.

To use, massage into dry or damp skin in a circular motion, then rinse with warm water and a cloth or muslin.

Spray the face and use a cotton wool pad with your choice of flower water to remove the last traces of the scrub.

EYE TREATMENT SERUM

It is important to take great care of the eye area as it is the most delicate and sensitive part of the skin, so only a small amount of a product is needed when applied to this region. As the eye area is typically a place of concern for fine lines and signs of ageing, this formula contains a trio of botanical oils renowned for their regenerative qualities, including meadowfoam oil to help prevent fine lines from developing.

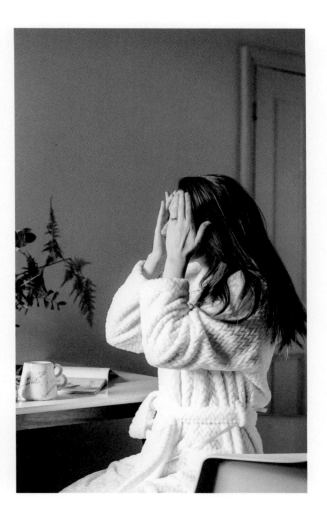

Ingredients

O   ⅓ teaspoon argan oil
O   ⅓ teaspoon meadowfoam oil
O   ⅓ teaspoon borage oil
O   ⅛ teaspoon vitamin E oil

Directions

Add the oils one by one into a clean 5-ml (⅙-fl oz) tinted glass bottle with a pipette top or roller ball dispenser. Shake gently to combine.

To use, glide the rollerball along the eye area very gently; if using a pipette, add one pipette of oil to each orbital bone.

Use the fingers to gently press the oil into the skin using a very light tapping motion, as if drawing imaginary spectacles around each eye. Use twice a day – morning and night.

MYRRH + NEROLI RICH HYDRATING MOISTURIZER

This recipe is for a basic hydrating cream or moisturizer which combines neroli flower water with rich nourishing oils, emulsifying wax and myrrh essential oil. Myrrh is a lesser-known treasure for skincare since it is a remarkable skin healer with outstanding regenerative and preservative properties, thus making it particularly valuable for damaged or mature skin types.

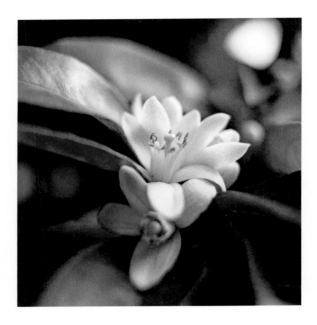

Ingredients

o   1 tablespoon emulsifying wax
o   4 teaspoons argan oil
o   3 teaspoons avocado oil
o   60 ml (2 fl oz) neroli flower water
o   12 drops myrrh essential oil

Directions

Place a glass jug or bowl over a small saucepan of water to create a bain-marie or use a double boiler. Bring the water to the boil and then reduce to a simmer. Add the emulsifying wax and oils to the jug or bowl and heat until the wax melts and turns liquid, stirring frequently. Place the neroli flower water in a heatproof beaker or Pyrex jug and stand this in the water to heat, but don't allow it to boil.

Once the emulsifying wax has melted, remove both items from the heat and combine them together, stirring for at least 2 minutes. Leave to stand for 1 minute, then stir again for 1 minute to ensure the blend becomes smooth in texture.

Repeat this process several times while the mixture cools. As it does so, it will thicken; once this begins to happen, add the myrrh essential oil and continue to stir to ensure it is distributed thoroughly into the lotion.

Once fully cooled and thickened, decant the lotion into an airtight tinted glass jar and use as within 4 weeks.

BEESWAX LIP + SKIN BALM

VEGAN LIP + SKIN BALM

Here is a lip balm recipe to keep the lips moisturized all day and to prevent them from cracking. The aim is to repair, rejuvenate, heal and deeply hydrate the lips to act as a preventative measure. The less calendula oil you add, the more solid the balm will become.

This lip balm omits the beeswax to make a vegan version and avoids including any animal products.

Ingredients

o   2 teaspoons solid coconut oil (or candelilla wax)
o   1 teaspoon shea butter
o   1 teaspoon avocado butter
o   3 tablespoons calendula oil

Ingredients

o   2 teaspoons beeswax
o   1 teaspoon shea butter
o   1 teaspoon avocado butter
o   3 tablespoons calendula oil

Directions

Combine all the ingredients in a 60-ml (2-fl oz) glass jar with a tight-fitting lid. Warm the shea butter a little beforehand if required. Stir with a glass rod until mixed well and combined.

To use, apply to lips or dry skin as required. Keep in the fridge for a firmer textured balm.

Directions

Combine all the ingredients in a 60-ml (2-fl oz) glass jar with a tight-fitting lid. Warm the shea butter a little beforehand if required. Stir with a glass rod until mixed well and combined.

To use, apply to lips or dry skin as required. Keep in the fridge for a firmer textured balm.

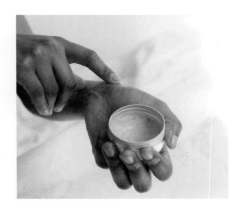

VARIATION

The ingredients are enough to make a 60-ml (2-fl oz) pot of balm, which can then be decanted into a smaller pot or jar, making it handy to keep in your bag over the summer, especially when the weather is hot.

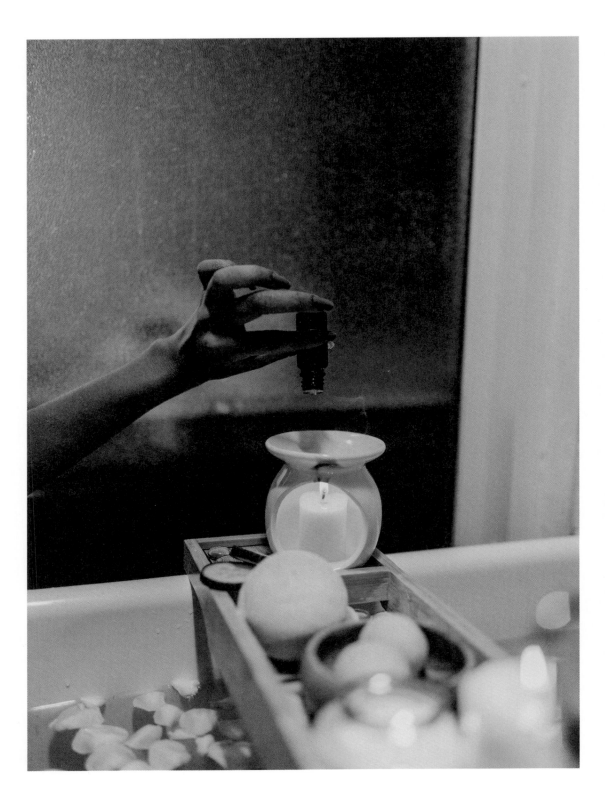

'Odours have a power of persuasion,
stronger than that of words, appearances,
emotions or will. The persuasive power of
an odour cannot be fended off, it enters into
us like breath into our lungs, it fills us up,
imbues us totally. There is no remedy for it.'

PATRICK SÜSKIND, *PERFUME*

4 + FRAGRANCE

Natural Perfumes + Home Fragrances

The power of scent is undeniable: the inhalation of a certain fragrance can immediately trigger a memory of a person or place and even transport us back to a location from our childhood. Perfumes have often been called the 'language of dreams' because they speak directly to our emotions in a subtle and often unconscious manner. In the 21st century, an era of science and technology, scent remains one of the last territories of the irrational. This is because our sense of smell is processed via the limbic system, also known as the emotional brain, which is beyond our logical control yet connects us directly to our primitive instincts.

When an odour is inhaled, it directly affects an area in our brain called the olfactory epithelium, which contains millions of tiny nerve endings. It is here that the fragrance is transmuted into a nerve message, which is amplified by the olfactory bulb, and then passed along the olfactory tract before enter-ing the limbic system. This part of the brain is also concerned with emotion

and related associations, so it is at this point that the odour may trigger a memory, either from a recent event or from the distant past. The message is then passed on to the hypothalamus, which acts as a relay station that sends it to other areas of the brain, so the effects are fully experienced.

But although these olfactory signals are processed by the so-called 'primitive' part of our brain, this does not imply that we are not being influenced by scent on a minute-to-minute basis – far from it! Our primal instincts, which function largely via our sense of smell, are alive and well, even if we are not generally aware of them. Today, we constantly try to cover up these life-preserving signals with a plethora of artificial smells and fragrances in our modern urban environment. Early societies, however, naturally valued and were keenly tuned in to these subliminal scent messages, both as a tool for survival – such as being able to ascertain whether a particular food was edible or not by its smell – as well as for more intimate indications, such as in choosing a sexual partner.

The early perfumes were all made from 100 per cent natural materials and could simultaneously serve as medicines, cosmetics or as ritual elixirs. These natural botanical ingredients were derived from flowers, aromatic roots, scented gums and spices, together with a small number of products derived from animals, such as musk. In early civilizations, natural aromatics and perfumes were highly valued as something essential and fundamental for preserving health and hygiene. But perfume was also regarded as something ritualistic and magical: a vital means by which to commune with the divine – a direct way to lift us out of our mundane existence to enjoy a sweet intoxication of the soul. Each culture naturally adopted their native species of flowers for their production of perfumes, such as jasmine and tuberose in India or lavender and frangipani in the Mediterranean. Perfumed woods such as sandalwood and cedarwood, which came from the East, together with a whole array of spices, such as cardamon, ginger and clove, gave the perfumes of the Orient a rich and sensual allure. Apart from their therapeutic value, scents were of course also used historically purely for aesthetic and sensual pleasure, much as they are today: jasmine and cardamon, for example, were considered to have aphrodisiac properties and were used to make love potions. But the scents of today are a

far cry from what they used to be in the ancient world, when there was little distinction made between medicine, incense and perfume.

Perfumes have been in use for over 8,000 years. Records suggest that the earliest perfumes were used in the East and Far East, especially within the ancient Chinese, Japanese and Indian cultures. In the Western world, the Egyptians were particularly renowned for their perfumery expertise, as were the ancient Greeks and Romans. The word 'perfume' literally means 'through the smoke' from the Latin *per fumare* since the smoking of fragrant plants and woods were the earliest type of perfumes. Incense and various forms of aromatic fumigations based on specific herbs were also commonly used to treat illness or to purify the air in religious ceremonies. This can still be seen in the traditional smudging ceremony of the Native Americans where smoke from the burning of white sage acts to cleanse a person, object or place from any negativity. In the Plains sweat lodge ritual, the floor of the structure is traditionally strewn with white sage leaves for the participants to inhale their fragrance and to rub on their bodies during the sweat. Likewise, in the sang ritual of the Tibetan and Himalayan cultures, the burning of plant materials such as cypress and juniper needles are used to purify both the individual and the environment.

Some early cultures and traditions were especially well versed in the psychoactive potentiality of aromatics. For example, the ancient Egyptians were renowned for their extraction of the rare blue lotus oil, which induced a pleasing, euphoric effect. The famous Egyptian perfume *kyphi* was made from a blend of 16 precious aromatic substances, including saffron, cinnamon, spikenard and calamus, which according to Plutarch, could 'lull one to sleep, allay anxiety and brighten dreams ... made of those things that delight most in the night'. The physician Marestheus also wrote of plants whose scents had an 'uplifting effect on the soul' such as the rose and hyacinth. Aromatics have traditionally been used to induce altered states of consciousness, both for lifting the spirits, as well as for driving out evil spirits in cases of mental illness. Frankincense, for example, has been employed as an incense for thousands of years due to its capacity to elevate the spirits and deepen the breath and is still used for its ritual effects in the Roman Catholic church. German research carried out in the 1980s demonstrated that the oleo-gum resin in frankincense contains a substance called tetrahydrocannabinol, related to cannabis oil, which has a mildly euphoric effect on the senses.

The first perfumes that were formulated to be applied to the skin were called unguents, a type of ointment made by simply immersing the aromatic material in an oily or fatty base. In ancient Egypt, these aromatic fatty perfumes were formed into cones and placed on the heads of the dancers at ritual events, so as they performed, the cones gradually melted, releasing their scent. Even

today, as part of an age-old ritual, a perfumed oil is used to anoint each newly enthroned British sovereign. The consecrated sacred formula used on the Coronation day of Elizabeth II in 1953 contained neroli, jasmine, rose, cinnamon, benzoin, musk, civet and ambergris in a base of sesame oil. The queen was anointed on the palms of her hands, her chest and her head as a central part of the ceremony. This ritual perfumed oil contained aromatics originally based on a Biblical recipe found in Exodus verse 30 using myrrh, cinnamon, cane and cassia in an olive oil base: 'Make these into a sacred anointing oil, a fragrant blend, the work of a perfumer. It will be the sacred anointing oil.'

The process of distillation of essential oils can be traced back thousands of years: clay pots used for distilling a primitive form of essential oil from plants have been discovered dating back to around 3,500 BCE in the Mesopotamian region. But it was only in the 11th century CE under the Arab physician Avicenna that this art was perfected. The Arab world enjoyed a passion for scent although they had different ingredients at their disposal. The Middle East is also said to have mastered the art of producing rose water, which is still an intrinsic part of their culture. It was from Arabia that knowledge of how to distil essential oils for making perfumes was first brought to medieval Europe. It is documented that European perfumers were subsequently largely immune from the plagues and infectious diseases that ravaged Europe at that time, since many essential oils exhibit potent anti-infectious and antiviral properties. Essential oils are especially effective as preventives against airborne infections because they vaporize naturally, as their biochemical name 'volatile oil' implies, and because they have an intrinsic affinity with the respiratory system when inhaled directly.

As the formulation and production of perfumes became more sophisticated, they took on a whole range of different forms to include scented powders, flower waters, eau-de-colognes, room fresheners as well as concentrated essences. Then, with the discovery of the alcoholic extraction process in the 14th century, the art of perfumery assumed a new finesse which was not previously possible using oily or fatty substances as the base material. The first books explaining perfumery techniques began to appear at the beginning of the early 16th century in Europe and it was common for large houses to prepare their own perfumes in a special 'still room', which contained a 'still', i.e., distillation apparatus.

The main purpose of the Elizabeth practice of drying and distilling herbs was initially for health and medicinal reasons, and secondarily for culinary purposes, such as the making of sweet-scented vinegar. The production of aromatic waters, perfumes, cosmetics, scented soaps and candles, moth repellents and potpourri, combined with making medicines, was a task traditionally carried out by the women of the household. Lavender and rose were extensively used for making fragrant waters, while furniture, writing paper and clothes were all scented with aromatic oils, such as cedarwood or patchouli; dried lavender flowers were also used to scent cloth and linen as a protection against moths.

It was not until the mid-19th century, however, that modern perfumery was born. Modern perfumes are distinct from those of their predecessors due to the discovery and employment of synthetic fragrances as opposed to those derived from natural materials. While herbs and natural aromatics have been used for thousands of years, synthetic scents only emerged some 150 years ago! And because synthetics can provide a limitless source of cheaper and more reliable notes, virtually all commercial perfumes found on the market today are made almost entirely from synthetics. An increasing number of people, however, are developing an adverse reaction or allergies to the mass of chemicals and toxic emissions with which we are surrounded in the modern world and are seeking out products which are 100 per cent natural. The growing interest in essential oils is therefore having a notable effect on the perfumery world with many cosmetic and perfumery houses now moving towards a more natural emphasis. Meanwhile, aromatherapy is moving in the direction of mainstream perfumery by becoming more sophisticated and far-reaching in its impact.

In classical perfumery, all fragrances are defined as having top notes, middle notes and base notes. Top notes are the scents which evaporate quickly, and include oils like mandarin, lime, bergamot and lemon; middle note fragrances form the body of the blend, with oils ranging from geranium, ylang-ylang to marjoram and clove; the base notes give a blend staying power or tenacity and include oils such as frankincense, sandalwood, benzoin or Peruvian balsam. In making natural perfumes, it is best to combine oils from all three categories to produce a balanced composition – this principle also generally applies when making blends for vaporization.

The art of perfumery is truly a form of alchemy! Even the smallest addition of a single drop of an essential oil can influence the overall balance of a composition. A perfume will also change over time – within seconds or in hours as each element evaporates – and the fragrance will naturally alter when it interacts with an individual's skin and body scent. This means that the same perfume will smell different on each person. There is an intimate connection between perfume and personality too, especially in relation to our basic drives of attraction and repulsion. We know that certain scents have the power to bring back long-forgotten memories, give pleasure or alternatively repel us, all on a subliminal level – but they can also effectively alter our mood, enhance our sense of wellbeing, uplift or soothe us.

In a series of experiments measuring the effect of specific essential oils on brainwave patterns using an electroencephalogram (EEG)

monitor, it was shown that scents can alter our brain wave patterns quite significantly, where an increase in alpha activity indicates a relaxing or soothing effect, whereas increased beta activity indicates increased levels of stimulation or attention. As a general rule in such studies, neroli, lavender, jasmine, rose, sandalwood, valerian, frankincense, chamomile and bergamot increased delta and alpha patterns, thereby slowing the mind's mental chatter, being similar to brain wave patterns induced by a meditative state. Whereas rosemary, basil, black pepper, cardamon, clove, peppermint and lemongrass increased beta activity, patterns characteristic of a state of arousal or alertness.

In addition, essential oils have been shown to affect brainwave patterns, inducing states of sedation or arousal, thus altering our mood simply via their fragrance. Training ourselves to become more sensitive and attuned to natural scents can help us connect to our intuition and instincts as well as to our emotional interior and needs.

Creating a sophisticated perfume that has many ingredients requires years of practice and expertise but making a simple pulse-point scent or a blend of essential oils for vaporization is very straightforward to do at home. Likewise, using herbs and aromatics to perfume cloth or furniture, as well as to make natural room fragrances and household aromatic products, is part of an age-old tradition that is easy, healthy and pleasurable to incorporate into our everyday routine.

PERFUME RECIPES

The art of perfumery is as old as civilization itself. It is a skill that requires precision and sensitivity, but above all the ability to translate an intangible idea into an actual composition. In the art of blending, balance is everything. The ideal perfume should be a perfect harmony between top, middle and base notes. When natural aromatic oils are combined, a chemical reaction occurs that breaks up their original molecular structure, so they recombine to form entirely new molecules ... a completely new perfume! The aim is to make a 'bouquet' or a 'seamless scent' where the whole adds up to more than just a sum of its parts. This is known as a 'synergy'. Before you begin, lay out all the ingredients and materials you need on a clean surface in an odour-free environment. You will need a selection of essential oils; jojoba oil or light coconut oil; a small, clean glass bottle with a roller, pipette or dropper top; a notepad and pen; glass stirring rod and some smelling strips. Assess the scent of each essential oil that you have selected in turn, then follow your intuition as to which proportions to use. Add the oils one drop at a time, as one drop can radically affect the overall balance. Don't forget to record the name and exact quantity of each oil you use at each stage of the blending process.

SOLID BODY PERFUMES

Solid perfumes are based on the ancient and original method for making body scents – known as 'unguents' – using oils and waxes as the base rather than alcohol, as is the case with most commercial perfumes produced today. It can be fun to experiment with making your own blends using the same basic process. These blends are safe to be applied to the body directly, such as to pulse points, on the neck or behind the ears. This type of perfume will have a very long shelf life of at least a year, as long as it is based on jojoba or light coconut oil.

'APHRODISIAC' PERFUME

Ingredients

- 1 teaspoon beeswax
- 1 teaspoon jojoba or light coconut oil
- 12 drops rose 5 per cent essential oil
- 12 drops sandalwood 5 per cent essential oil
- 4 drops ylang ylang essential oil
- 4 drops cardamon essential oil
- 3 drops patchouli essential oil
- 3 drops lime essential oil

'FOREST' (UNISEX) PERFUME

Ingredients

- 1 teaspoon beeswax
- 1 teaspoon jojoba or light coconut oil
- 10 drops vetiver essential oil
- 10 drops cedarwood essential oil
- 5 drops elemi essential oil
- 5 drops juniper needle essential oil
- 5 drops cypress essential oil
- 5 drops pine essential oil

'INNER PEACE' PERFUME

Ingredients

- 1 teaspoon beeswax
- 1 teaspoon jojoba or light coconut oil
- 10 drops bergamot essential oil
- 10 drops ho leaf essential oil
- 8 drops rose geranium essential oil
- 8 drops clary sage essential oil
- 2 drops clove essential oil

Directions

Place a glass bowl over a small saucepan of water to create a bain-marie or use a double boiler. Bring to the boil, then reduce to a simmer.

Add the beeswax and, once melted, add the jojoba or light coconut oil. Once the oil has turned to a liquid, pour into a glass jar or aluminium tin.

Add the essential oils one by one and stir gently using a glass rod for 30 seconds to combine. Leave to set for 30 minutes before using.

ROOM FRAGRANCE DIFFUSER BLENDS

Using essential oils in an essential oil diffuser has become very popular in recent years. There is now a vast array of traditional oil burners as well as many types of electric diffusers available, some which are also room humidifiers. The electric diffusers have the advantage of being much safer to use, especially around children or pets, as they do not have a live flame. It is a good idea to choose a diffuser that suits the size of your home and workplace then use it regularly, as vaporizing essential oils is an excellent way to not only scent a space naturally, but also to prevent the spread of any unwelcome airborne bacteria. This type of room fragrance will have a very long shelf life of at least two years, as long as it is based on pure essential oils.

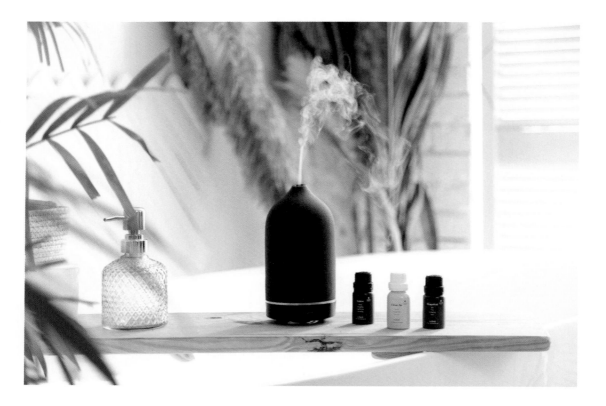

'UPLIFT' ROOM FRAGRANCE

Ingredients

- 60 drops orange essential oil
- 40 drops peppermint essential oil
- 80 drops bergamot essential oil
- 20 drops lime essential oil

'MEDITATE' ROOM FRAGRANCE

Ingredients

- 50 drops elemi essential oil
- 50 drops myrrh essential oil
- 25 drops frankincense essential oil
- 25 drops patchouli essential oil
- 50 drops grapefruit essential oil

'PREVENT' ROOM FRAGRANCE

Ingredients

- 60 drops basil essential oil
- 40 drops thyme essential oil
- 60 drops ravensara essential oil
- 40 drops lime essential oil

'SLEEP' ROOM FRAGRANCE

Ingredients

- 60 drops lavender essential oil
- 60 drops petitgrain essential oil
- 40 drops vetiver essential oil
- 40 drops cedarwood essential oil

Directions

Add the essential oils one by one to a tinted glass 10-ml (⅓-fl oz) bottle with a pipette lid. Place the lid on to secure and shake well to combine.

Add 6–10 drops to an electric diffuser or oil burner each time you want to enjoy the fragrance.

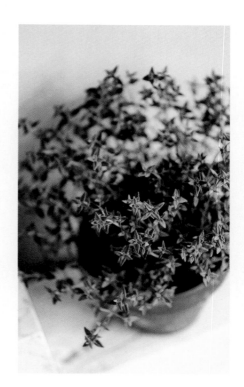

LIGHT PERFUME HOUSEHOLD MISTS

These light perfume mists are based on flower waters further infused with natural essential oils. They make lovely refreshing room fragrances, which can also be used to perfume clothes, linen and furniture. This type of lightweight room fragrance will have a very long shelf life of at least a year, as long as it is based on pure flower waters and essential oils.

For light perfumes that are to be applied to the body, use the blended flower water recipes found in the skincare section under toners, as these can also be sprayed directly onto the skin as a fragrant aqua spritz.

'LOVE POTION' PERFUME MIST

Spray around your surroundings, such as the living area and the bedroom. Please note that this blend contains vegetable oils so may stain clothes or linen; patch test before use.

Ingredients

- 2 teaspoons witch hazel water
- 15 drops jasmine 5 per cent essential oil
- 15 drops sandalwood 5 per cent essential oil
- 10 drops rose maroc 5 per cent essential oil
- 10 drops cardamom essential oil
- 90 ml (3 fl oz) rose water

'FRESH PERSPECTIVE' YOGA MIST

Spray the mist onto your yoga mat or around the room or studio before and after practice.

Ingredients

- 2 teaspoons witch hazel water
- 20 drops palmarosa essential oil
- 20 drops petitgrain essential oil
- 10 drops peppermint essential oil
- 90 ml (3 fl oz) fragonia water

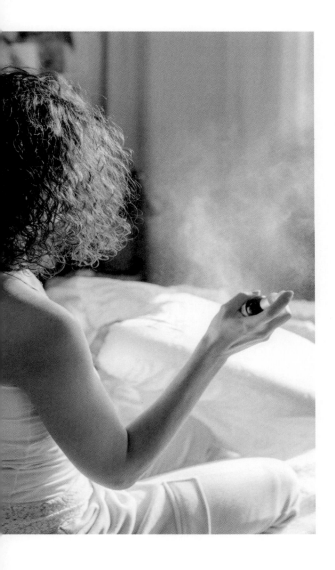

'SLEEP' PILLOW MIST

Spray onto pillows, nightwear
and around the bedroom.

Ingredients

- o 2 teaspoons witch hazel water
- o 15 drops lavender essential oil
- o 15 drops neroli essential oil
- o 10 drops clary sage essential oil
- o 10 drops vetiver essential oil
- o 90 ml (3 fl oz) lavender water

'CREATIVITY' DESKSIDE MIST

Spray around your desk or workspace
or whenever you want to inspire
creativity.

Ingredients

- o 2 teaspoons witch hazel water
- o 15 drops rosemary essential oil
- o 15 drops basil essential oil
- o 10 drops mandarin essential oil
- o 10 drops grapefruit essential oil
- o 90 ml (3 fl oz) rosemary water

Directions

Add the witch hazel to a 15-ml
(½-fl oz) tinted glass bottle with an
atomizer spray top. Next, add the
essential oils one by one, and finish
with the flower water. Place the
atomizer top on the bottle and give it
a good shake. It is ready to use and
enjoy immediately.

TRADITIONAL POTPOURRI BLEND

Making potpourri is fun, especially for children – it can be an endlessly creative exercise since virtually any kind of dried natural materials can be included. The recipe here is based on classic potpourri ingredients, but I like to dry any leaves, petals or other types of plant material, such as small fir cones or seed heads – anything that has a nice texture, colour or scent – then combine them together with essential oils to display in a decorative bowl. Plant materials can be easily prepared at home by laying them out on newspaper to dry. Potpourri was originally created in the 12th century for the purpose of freshening the air within the home, especially on wealthy estates, since spices and herbs were the principal means of keeping the house hygienic and free of airborne germs.

Ingredients

- ¼ nutmeg, grated
- ½ tablespoon orris root powder
- 10 drops rose essential oil
- 30 drops lavender essential oil
- 10 drops lime essential oil
- 2 cups dried rose petals
- ½ cup dried lavender flowers
- ½ cup dried verbena leaves

Directions

Grind the grated nutmeg and orris root powder together in a pestle and mortar, then add half the total quantity of essential oils and mix using a spoon or glass rod.

Next place the main dried plant ingredients in a glass or ceramic sealable storage container and add the remaining essential oils, mixing well. Add the powdered material from the mortar and mix gently so as not to damage the botanical materials.

Seal the container and leave to mature for 2 to 6 weeks in a dark place.

Transfer the potpourri mixture into a decorative bowl or jar. Later, as the aroma starts to fade, more essential oils can be added to revive the mixture and prolong its life.

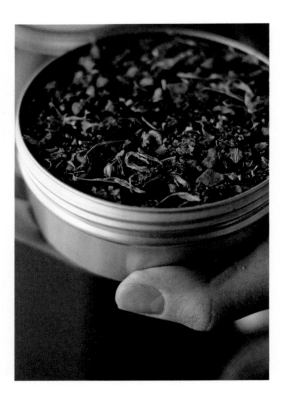

PULSE-POINT ROLLERBALL PERFUMES

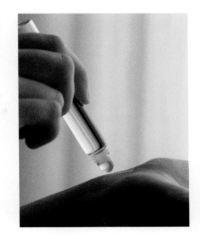

These pulse-point rollerball scents are based on herbal or vegetable oils rather than waxes, as is the case with the original unguent-style perfumes. They are very versatile to use and easy to carry with you while you are out and about, good for some self-help on the move. Those recipes based on infused herbal oils will have a shelf life of approximately 6 months, while those based on light coconut oil will last for up to two years.

'EMOTIONAL CRISIS SUPPORT' PERFUME

Ingredients

- 2 teaspoons St John's wort oil
- 6 drops rose essential oil
- 3 drops marjoram essential oil
- 2 drops frankincense essential oil
- 2 drops cypress essential oil

'SELF-ESTEEM BOOST' PERFUME

Ingredients

- 2 teaspoons calendula-infused oil
- 6 drops jasmine essential oil
- 3 drops neroli essential oil
- 2 drops rose essential oil
- 2 drops patchouli essential oil

'FOCUS + CONCENTRATE' PERFUME

Ingredients

- 2 teaspoons light coconut oil
- 4 drops rosemary essential oil
- 3 drops geranium essential oil
- 3 drops sweet orange essential oil
- 2 drops black pepper essential oil

Directions

Add the oil to clean 10-ml (⅓-fl oz) rollerball bottle. Add the essential oils one by one. Place the roller ball and cap on and shake well to combine. It is ready to use immediately.

To use, apply to your pulse points, massage into the soles of the feet or rub beneath the nostrils, and take 10 deep, expansive breaths using the scent as an anchor.

BATHROOM / TOILET DROP AIR-FRESHENERS

To keep your bathroom smelling fragrant, fresh and clean, these formulations provide a natural solution. The recipes are all based on pure essential oils and provide an extra boost of airborne aromatic hygiene to your bathroom due to their potent antiseptic and bactericidal properties. Simply blend all the ingredients together – it's important to leave them to mature for 24 hours – then remember to label each one well and keep a bottle handy in your bathroom beside the toilet for daily use. Each blend will last for a year or more.

'SPRING' AIR FRESHENER

Ingredients

- 2 teaspoons rubbing alcohol
- 50 drops pine essential oil
- 50 drops grapefruit essential oil
- 50 drops lemon essential oil
- 50 drops peppermint essential oil
- 90 ml (3 fl oz) witch hazel water

'SUMMER' AIR FRESHENER

Ingredients

- 2 teaspoons rubbing alcohol
- 50 drops ylang ylang essential oil
- 50 drops geranium essential oil
- 50 drops palmarosa essential oil
- 50 drops basil essential oil
- 90 ml (3 fl oz) witch hazel water

'AUTUMN' AIR FRESHENER

Ingredients

- 2 teaspoons rubbing alcohol
- 50 drops cedarwood essential oil
- 50 drops cypress essential oil
- 50 drops bergamot essential oil
- 50 drops black pepper essential oil
- 90 ml (3 fl oz) witch hazel water

'WINTER' AIR FRESHENER

Ingredients

- 2 teaspoons rubbing alcohol
- 50 drops clove essential oil
- 50 drops cinnamon essential oil
- 50 drops mandarin essential oil
- 50 drops ginger essential oil
- 90 ml (3 fl oz) witch hazel water

4+ Fragrance

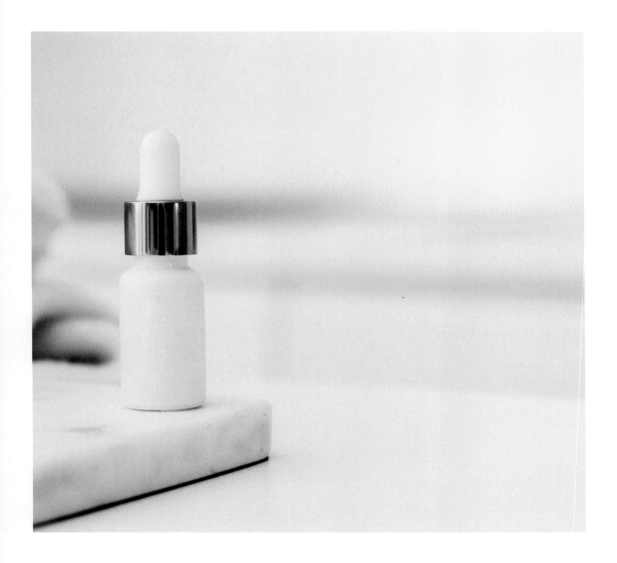

Directions

Add the rubbing alcohol to a clean
100-ml (3½-fl oz) glass pipette bottle.
Add the essential oils one by one, then
top up with the witch hazel water.
Leave for 24 hours to mature.

To use, add 1–2 pipettes to the toilet
pan for each use.

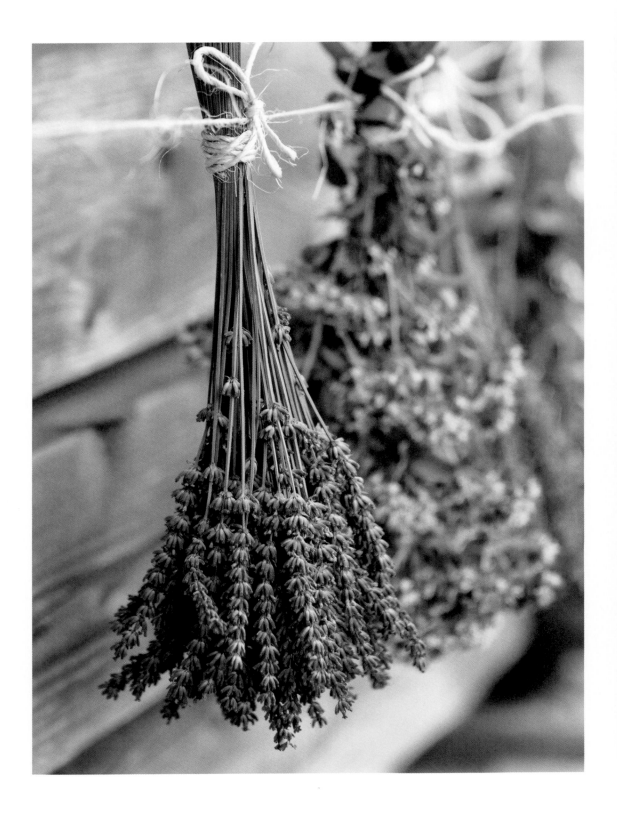

'Mama's most important herb was parsley, which along with dill, marjoram, hops and others were dried in bunches in the autumn, dangling at the end of short lengths of cotton, all strung on a long length of thin rope, stretching right across the kitchen stove.'

JULIA LAWLESS, *THE ENCYCLOPEDIA OF ESSENTIAL OILS*

5 + MEDICINE

First Aid, Herbs, Oils + Ointments

Herbs and essential oils have long been used at home as first aid remedies for common complaints; these were once known as herbal 'simples'. This includes the treatment of skin conditions like burns, cuts, bruises and boils, as well as many other common problems, such as headaches or digestive upsets. Many respiratory complaints such as coughs, colds and flu also respond well to treatment using essential oils via the simple technique of steam inhalation because they vaporize readily. At one time it was commonplace to apply many of these simple remedies at home, in the form of herbal salves, oils and ointments, but over the last century the knowledge of how to use these traditional remedies has largely been lost in the West. This is not the case in Finland, however, where a more intimate connection with nature has remained intact.

I was named after my Finnish grandmother who was called Julia, but generally she was simply known as Mama. Both my grandmother and my mother Kerttu were well versed in

the use of herbs and would grow a number of aromatic plants specifically for their medicinal usage. My mother's family came from Rauma in the south-west of Finland, which today is a UNESCO world heritage site. Situated on the Gulf of Bothnia, Rauma is one of few remaining medieval towns in Finland made up of traditional wooden buildings, most having inner paved courtyards with decorative gates within which herbs and other plants could be grown sheltered from the harsh winter conditions. Mama would grow a variety of herbs within the cobbled courtyard and then dry her favourite ones to make remedies for use over the winter months, using plants such as parsley, dill, hops and marjoram. These would then be hung to dry on string above the kitchen stove or on wooden poles across the ceiling of her long, narrow storage room, together with her flat, dry rye bread.

Herbs and aromatic materials have traditionally played an intrinsic role in the daily practices of most cultures, especially for the maintenance of health and hygiene since plants were the most potent medicinal substances available. Aromatics such as frankincense, myrrh and a whole array of spices, were therefore some of the most important substances in the ancient world, where whole trade routes were based on their transportation around the globe. Precious spices such as cloves and black pepper were not just culinary aids but also used to ward off infection, while myrrh was used not only as an incense material, but also as a wound healing salve. Roman soldiers were even required to carry a phial of myrrh with them onto the battlefield as a hands-on first aid remedy in case of injury. Scientific research is now confirming many of the traditional usages of aromatics as well as making new and valuable discoveries. For example, it has now been found that essential oils interact with our own biological cellular activity in such a way that makes them very effective healing agents on a basic molecular level.

The practice of using botanical aromatics for first aid purposes and as natural remedies benefits from being placed within the context of naturopathic healthcare as a whole – from a holistic point of view, the best form of treatment is always a multifaceted one. Exercise, diet, sleep and relaxation as well as our emotional and mental disposition are all essential factors which need to be taken into account when we are considering the treatment of any common complaint. It is also vital to consider preventative medicine as

a very important part of the holistic approach – something that Western medicine does not always fully appreciate. When we use essential oils and natural aromatics as part of our daily routine for bathing, skincare, massage, perfumes and as remedies for common complaints, then we naturally tend to have a higher level of resistance to illness, catching fewer colds on average and recovering more quickly when we do become sick. This is because many aromatic herbs and essential oils exhibit potent anti-infectious and antiviral properties, thus supporting the immune system.

The immune response is orchestrated by three distinct groups of cells, the phagocytes, the 'T' cells and the 'B' cells. These all originate from white blood cells in the bone marrow and serve to protect the body from infection. If this defensive barrier is damaged for some reason, the body becomes more vulnerable to invasion from all sorts of pathogenic organisms. The immune system is supported by and closely related to other body functions including the lymphatic and nervous systems. Recent research tends to suggest that emotional and psychological factors play a vital role in the efficiency of the immune response, and this may help to account for the fact that viral infections and suppressed immune systems are becoming an increasing problem today.

Maintaining a relaxed state of mind is therefore central to supporting the immune system naturally, as part of a larger preventative approach to disease. When we are stressed, the amygdala is activated, which puts our body into a 'fight or flight' mode increasing glucose in our system – but if this is switched on all the time it causes stress, anxiety and lack of sleep. Recent research at Harvard University in Massachusetts has demonstrated that the opposite to the stress response can be activated through yoga, meditation or prayer. All these practises slow the breathing and thus can help to control anxiety or fear. The study also suggested that meditation can help replace the loss of telomerase, a key enzyme which encourages cellular regeneration; so regular meditation and yoga can help slow the ageing process and increase cellular regeneration, as well as keep the immune system strong.

Today, there are many essential oils available from across the world which can help to support our immune system naturally, such as tea tree, fragonia, lemon eucalyptus, lemon myrtle, rosemary, thyme and ravintsara, all of which been shown to exhibit powerful bactericidal activity, which assists the body in resisting and fighting infection. One of the disadvantages of extracting isolated active ingredients for the treatment of infection, such as cineole, which is commonly used in pharmaceutical cough medicines – the principal active constituent found in eucalyptus oil – is that pathogens can find ways of building up resistance to this single isolate. By contrast, the complex biochemical composition of essential oils makes them very resistant to pathogens which is valuable in those

cases where resistance has built up to conventional treatments such as antibiotics, as is becoming increasingly common. There are many factors which can lead to a damaged immune system, such as stress or over-exposure to chemical toxins and pollution, but notably the over-use of antibiotics. Insecticides and the many synthetic additives found in our food and cosmetics can also contribute to the breakdown of our natural immunity.

There are also several essential oils that help build up our natural immunity by specifically supporting the respiratory system, such as frankincense, sandalwood and myrrh. Respiratory conditions, such as coughs, colds and flu as well as airborne infections respond extremely well to the use of essential oils simply through the process of inhalation. When we breathe in the aromatic vapours of a particular oil, the active therapeutic properties of that plant are readily absorbed by the mucus membranes lining the whole respiratory tract, including the lungs. This can be achieved via steam inhalation, or by simply inhaling the oil (or a blend of oils) directly using a room diffuser or vaporizer.

Perhaps the three most valuable essential oils to have at home in an aromatic medicine chest, as well to take with you when travelling, are tea tree, lavender and rosemary. Tea tree oil especially has been subjected to a great deal of scientific research in the last few decades regarding its bactericidal and antiviral properties plus its ability to support the immune system. For example, in an experiment carried out in Australia in 1980, tea tree oil was found to be an effective germicide at only four parts essential oil to 1,000 parts water. In another trial in 1983, it was found that tea tree oil reduced the bacteria count on hands from 3,000 per 50 cm (20 in) to 3 per 50 cm. The effectiveness of tea tree oil in fighting infection is further backed up by its ability to stimulate the immune system, that is, tea tree oil increases the body's own capacity to protect itself and respond defensively. In some hospitals, tea tree oil is already being used to help increase the immune response of patients waiting for surgery and aid recovery of those with long-term debilitating illnesses. What makes tea tree remarkable is that the oil is active against all three types of infectious organisms: bacteria, fungi and viruses. Tea tree oil is also useful in combatting feverish conditions associated with viral infection, used in vaporizers and steam inhalations. In addition, tea tree water is ideal for general household disinfectant use, for hands and for cleaning surfaces. However, tea tree oil has a strong medicinal smell which some people find off-putting – it can also cause skin sensitization or irritation in some individuals: if this is the case, fragonia oil makes an excellent substitute.

Lavender is perhaps the most versatile home remedy used in aromatherapy and by far the most popular essential oil. Lavender oil has a relaxing, familiar scent and can help aid sleep by just adding a few drops to an evening bath. It can also help ease stressful states of mind simply through inhalation: it is now being used in vaporizers in some hospitals to help patients overcome anxiety or worrying thoughts, aid sleep and to create a calm atmosphere. Very soothing when applied to the skin, lavender helps minor cuts and wounds to heal rapidly, easing pain and helping to prevent scarring. Lavender oil is one of the few oils that can be applied neat to the skin: for example, a few drops can be applied directly to burns, bumps, insect bites, rashes or spots. Lavender oil also brings relief from muscular aches and pains applied locally in combination with massage or used on a compress to reduce swelling: the compress can either be cold or hot depending on the condition. Lavender flowers have also traditionally been used to scent linen or pillowcases to encourage sleep.

Rosemary is a very valuable essential oil to keep in the home medicine kit. The oil has a lovely, fresh-green, stimulating scent that makes the mind instantly feel more alert – good while studying or for promoting concentration. Rosemary is also excellent for soothing general aches and pains or stiffness, especially in combination with lavender oil. It is one of the most important oils to combat any type of contagious airborne infection: for example, it can help prevent colds and coughs from developing at the very beginning due to its potent anti-infectious and antiviral properties. Used in vaporizers in the home, workplace or office it can help prevent the spread of germs, viruses and airborne infection.

In Europe during the 16th century, rosemary was burned in public places to help contain the Great Plague and was carried by individuals in special pouches while travelling. The secret aromatic recipe, used by the so-called 'four thieves' to combat the plague epidemic while stealing from the ill, is known to have consisted of cinnamon, cloves, camphor, eucalyptus, rosemary and lemon. All these essential oils were subsequently tested at Weber State University (Utah) in 1997 and found to have 99.96 per cent effectiveness against airborne bacteria. These aromatics are still among the most effective oils for protecting against airborne contagious infections.

Today there are also many other essential oils such as bergamot, grapefruit, lemon or lime, which can be used in vaporizers to purify the air, creating a fresh, uplifting feeling while disinfecting the environment naturally. According to modern scientific research, lemon eucalyptus, may chang and lemongrass, which all contain high amounts of citral or citronellal, exhibit good antimicrobial activity, while juniper berry, thyme and pine oil exhibit excellent bactericidal properties. Other camphoraceous essential oils that have valuable anti-infectious properties include eucalyptus, ravintsara, ravensara, cajeput and niaouli – good for respiratory problems and clearing congestion. All the spice oils help to bring heat to our whole metabolism thereby supporting the entire system by helping to combat chills alongside powerful antiseptic, bactericidal and antiviral properties. Oils such as clove, cinnamon leaf, black pepper, ginger and cardamom therefore make potent additions to therapeutic blends for vaporization, added in small amounts. It is worthwhile to invest in an efficient electric diffuser in times of contagious disease to help combat the spread of germs and to support the immune and respiratory system naturally.

Just a few ingredients from your first aid kit will enable you to treat many common complaints at home, such as headaches, period pains or digestive upsets, and enable you to make simple balms, creams and ointments which can be used to treat minor injuries, such as gardening scrapes, cuts, insect bites or sunburn. Salves, ointments, and balms are prepared from a mix of fatty ingredients such as oils and waxes, usually with no water at all. This differentiates them from creams and lotions which contain both fats and water. Suitable ingredients for making this form of preparation include vegetable oils such as sweet almond oil, apricot oil or jojoba oil combined with beeswax or a vegetable wax such as candelilla. It is therefore very useful to build up a basic medicine kit for home use – also invaluable when you are travelling abroad – of the most useful essential oils, together with a few of the most important carrier oils, to always have on hand. A few herbs are also vital, such as calendula for treating wounds and aloe vera for its cooling properties, as well as different types of clay for making poultices and shea butter for making salves – include these in your home medicine cabinet.

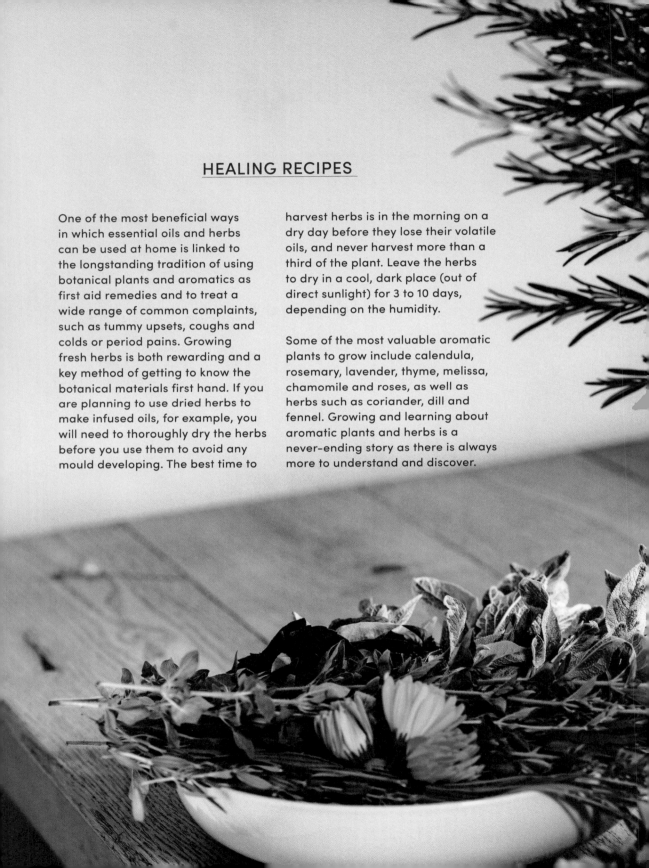

HEALING RECIPES

One of the most beneficial ways in which essential oils and herbs can be used at home is linked to the longstanding tradition of using botanical plants and aromatics as first aid remedies and to treat a wide range of common complaints, such as tummy upsets, coughs and colds or period pains. Growing fresh herbs is both rewarding and a key method of getting to know the botanical materials first hand. If you are planning to use dried herbs to make infused oils, for example, you will need to thoroughly dry the herbs before you use them to avoid any mould developing. The best time to harvest herbs is in the morning on a dry day before they lose their volatile oils, and never harvest more than a third of the plant. Leave the herbs to dry in a cool, dark place (out of direct sunlight) for 3 to 10 days, depending on the humidity.

Some of the most valuable aromatic plants to grow include calendula, rosemary, lavender, thyme, melissa, chamomile and roses, as well as herbs such as coriander, dill and fennel. Growing and learning about aromatic plants and herbs is a never-ending story as there is always more to understand and discover.

HEALING CALENDULA INFUSED OIL

Herbal infused oils make great bases for balms, salves and massage oils. They can also be added to a warm bath or simply used to soothe common skin problems, such as rashes, dermatitis and mild sunburn. Calendula is one of the most valuable herbs for healing the skin, especially for bruised or sore areas. While there is no exact science on the oil to herb ratio in an infused oil, the aim is to completely cover the plant material with oil. The advantage of using light coconut or jojoba oil as the menstruum or solvent is that these do not go rancid with age. Other vegetable oils, such as sweet almond, grapeseed or apricot kernel oil, may also be used but their shelf life will be shorter.

Ingredients

○ 2 tablespoons dried calendula flowers (or other herbs)
○ 200 ml (7 fl oz) coconut or jojoba oil (or alternative carrier oils)

Directions

Place your dried herbs in a clean, sterilized glass jar, then cover them with the oil and seal. Leave on a sunny windowsill for roughly 4 weeks to infuse, giving the jar a little shake every few days.

After 4 weeks, strain the herbs and pour into a clean, tinted glass bottle and seal. Don't discard the herbs: you can rub the flowers or herbs directly on the skin as they will still be covered in nourishing, replenishing goodness, or add them to a bath.

To use, apply the infused oil directly to the skin or use it in the skin, bath and body recipes in this book.

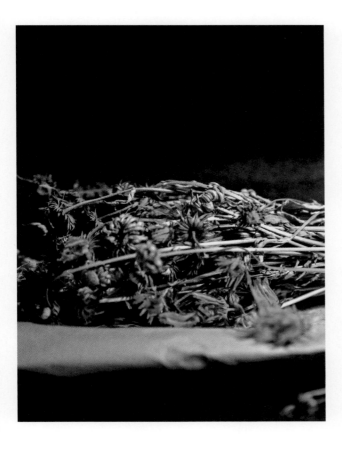

VARIATION

Comfrey, St John's wort and lavender also make excellent infused oils. You can either grow your own herbs and use them fresh, dry them yourself or buy dried herbs.

COOLING HERBAL COMPRESS

ESSENTIAL OIL COLD COMPRESS

Herbal tisanes or herbal tea bags of chamomile or elderflower make ideal compresses which can be applied to tired eyes as well as to itchy, inflamed or sensitive skin. They can also be placed on the area around swollen eyes for hay fever, styes or conjunctivitis. It is best to cool the wet tea bags first by placing them in the fridge – or if you are using home-grown herbs, to wrap them securely in wet muslin – then apply when needed.

Ingredients

o   2 teaspoons dried chamomile or elderflower (or 2 tea bags)
o   Boiled water

Directions

Infuse the dried chamomile flowers or elderflower (or herbal tea bags) in a mug of boiled water. Allow it to cool, then place it in the fridge.

Once cooled, wrap the herbs in two muslin squares, tie securely, and apply to closed eyes or the affected area for immediate relief; alternatively apply the teabags directly.

A cold compress using essential oils is very valuable in cases of localized inflammation due to minor injuries, such as sprains or muscular aches and pains, and also for insect bites or sunburn. Lavender and chamomile are both soothing herbs which will reduce swelling and relieve pain.

Ingredients

o   1 cup cold water
o   2 drops chamomile essential oil
o   2 drops lavender essential oil
o   Small flannel (washcloth)

Directions

Add 1 cup of cold water to a small bowl. Add the essential oils and agitate the water. Soak a flannel in the cold water. Apply to the affected area for 1 minute. Repeat several times for immediate relief.

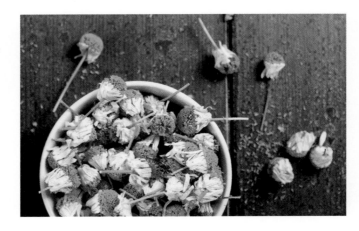

TEA TREE OIL + CLAY WARM POULTICE

A clay poultice is useful to help draw poisons or toxins out of the skin in the case of boils, stings or bites – and for cleaning dirty wounds – and the honey and chamomile have a soothing effect. Tea tree essential oil is very effective in preventing pus or any infection developing. This poultice is best employed fresh but can be refrigerated in an airtight container for up to a week.

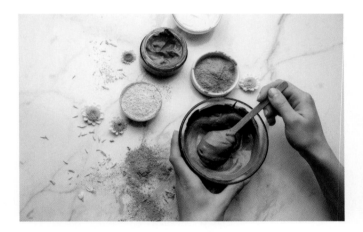

Ingredients

○ 60 grams (2 oz) bentonite clay
○ ½ cup of warm chamomile herbal tea
○ 2 drops tea tree essential oil
○ 1 tablespoon manuka honey (optional)
○ Muslin or gauze square and medical tape

Directions

Whisk or stir the clay, chamomile tea, tea tree oil and honey, if using, together in a small bowl.

To use, apply the warm clay poultice liberally to a square of gauze or muslin. Adhere the gauze poultice to the skin, covering the boil or bite, using tape to secure, if needed. Leave in place for two to three hours before removing.

Upon removing the poultice, cleanse the skin well and dress the wound accordingly. Repeat two to three times a day or as required.

ROSE + GLYCERINE LOTION

Rose and glycerine make a traditional remedy to soothe the heart and treat stress-related complaints such as anxiety and depression. Our skin can flare up when we are under pressure or emotionally upset and this soothing and moisturizing lotion can help bring relief.

Ingredients

o   At least 50 grams (1¾ oz) fresh rose petals
o   100 ml (3½ fl oz) vegetable glycerine

Directions

Pack a clean sterilized glass jar with your fresh rose petals. Pour the glycerine over the fresh herbs to fill the jar and seal tightly. Shake well to make sure the herbs are completely covered.

Leave to infuse for 5 to 6 weeks, remembering to shake the jar every day. Strain out the herbs and store in a dark tinted glass bottle.

To use, apply the remedy directly to the skin or add to any face, body, massage or bath blends in this book. Best used within 12 months.

ALOE VERA SOOTHING SKIN GEL

Aloe vera gel is cooling, soothing and anti-inflammatory – it also combines well with essential oils for first aid purposes, especially for calming the skin in cases of dermatitis, heat rash and itchy skin complaints. It is also valuable for treating inflamed skin caused by insect bites or sunburn.

Ingredients

o   50 ml (1¾ fl oz) aloe vera gel
o   15 drops lavender essential oil
o   15 drops chamomile essential oil

Directions

Add the aloe vera gel to a 500-ml (16-fl oz) tinted glass jar. Add the essential oil drops one at a time. Stir well with a glass rod and seal the top.

Use immediately by applying direct to skin. Best used within 6 months.

VARIATION

For a single-use application, combine 1 teaspoon aloe vera with 1 drop each of lavender and chamomile essential oils.

AFTER-SUN SOOTHING LAVENDER MIST

This makes an excellent mist for the face and body after hot days spent outdoors and it helps soothe the complexion and prevents any redness or soreness developing. Prevention is always better than cure! Aloe vera is naturally cooling, witch hazel water helps close the pores, glycerine is moisturizing, and lavender is renowned for its skin-healing properties, especially as a remedy for burns and abrasions.

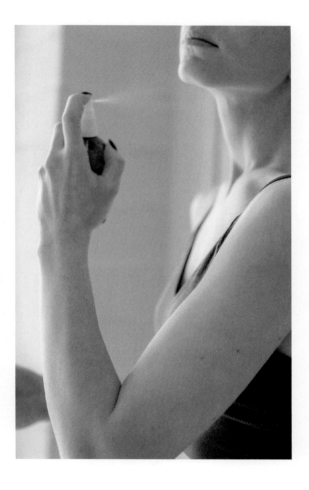

Ingredients

○ 2 teaspoons witch hazel
○ 1 tablespoon vegetable glycerine
○ 1 tablespoon aloe vera water or gel
○ 60 ml (2 fl oz) lavender water
○ 10 drops lavender essential oil

Directions

Add the ingredients, one by one in the order above, to a 100-ml (3½-fl oz) tinted glass bottle with atomizer top. Place the atomizer on top, close tightly and give the bottle a good shake. For optimum refreshment, keep it cool in the fridge.

Shake well before each use and spray liberally onto face and body as required. Use within 6 months.

SCAR + STRETCH MARK OIL

Argan oil enriched with vitamin E (or wheatgerm oil) increases the elasticity and regeneration of the skin, so massaging it onto scars or stretch marks helps heal the broken tissues gradually making the marks fade. This recipe also includes myrrh and rose essential oil together with borage oil and 'carrot' (or algae) infused oil for their remarkable restorative properties. Ideally however, it is best to prevent stretch marks from occurring beforehand by lubricating the skin liberally with this oil recipe during the last 4 months of pregnancy (see also the Safety Guidelines on page 168).

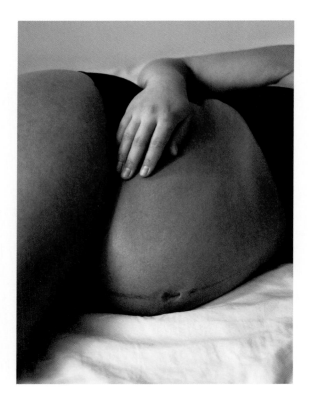

Ingredients

- 80 ml (2¾ fl oz) argan oil
- 2 teaspoons borage oil
- 1 teaspoon 'carrot' (algae) oil
- 1 teaspoon vitamin E oil (or wheatgerm oil)
- 10 drops myrrh essential oil
- 10 drops rose essential oil

Directions

Add the carrier oils one by one to a clean 100-ml (3½-fl oz) tinted glass bottle with a pump top. Add in the drops of essential oil one by one. Place the pump lid on the bottle, close tightly and shake well.

Apply to the skin as needed.

5+ Medicine

NAPPY RASH BALM

This is a 100 per cent natural gentle recipe for soothing nappy rash for children over 6 months old. For newborn babies, the essential oils must be omitted from the recipe.

Ingredients

- 1 tablespoon calendula oil
- 1 tablespoon peach or apricot kernel oil
- 1 tablespoon cocoa, shea or aloe vera butter (optional)
- 2 teaspoons beeswax
- 2 drops chamomile essential oil
- 2 drops lavender essential oil
- 2 drops fragonia essential oil

Directions

Place a glass jug or bowl over a small saucepan of water to create a bain-marie or use a double boiler. Bring the water to the boil and then reduce to a simmer. Add the carrier oils, butter, if using, and the beeswax. Keep on the heat until everything has melted, stirring regularly.

Remove from the heat and add the essential oils one by one. Stir well with a spoon or glass rod.

Pour the balm mix into a glass jar or aluminium tin and allow the mix to set for approximately 20 minutes.

Once set, it is ready to use. Apply once a day, or as required.

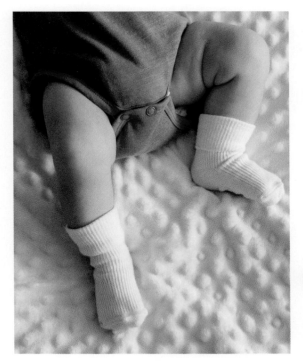

LIFESTYLE TIP

Instead of light talcum powder, use colloidal oatmeal to soothe irritation or redness on your baby's skin.

HEADACHE RELIEF BALM

Lavender is a classic remedy for headaches and migraine – here it is combined with peppermint for an extra cooling effect.

Ingredients

- 50 ml (1¾ fl oz) coconut or sweet almond oil
- 2 teaspoons beeswax
- 10 drops peppermint essential oil
- 10 drops lavender essential oil

Directions

Place a glass jug or bowl over a small saucepan of water to create a bain-marie or use a double boiler. Bring the water to the boil and then reduce to a simmer. Add the carrier oil and beeswax to the jug or bowl and heat until everything has melted, stirring regularly.

Remove from the heat, add the essential oils and stir with a glass rod to combine. Pour the mixture into a tinted glass jar and allow to set for 10 to 15 minutes, then seal.

Use immediately or keep in the fridge for a firmer textured balm.

To soothe headaches and tension in the neck area, apply to the temples, forehead and back of the neck.

OIL RUB FOR PMS / PAINFUL PERIODS

This oil blend is best applied right after a bath or shower when the skin is warm and rubbed gently into the abdomen in a clockwise circle. This recipe is enough for no more than a couple of applications, in which case St John's wort oil can be used. You can also increase the proportions if you wish to make a larger batch if it is a recurrent issue; for larger amounts, it is best to use light coconut or jojoba oil as they do not deteriorate with age.

Ingredients

- 2 teaspoons St John's wort oil (or light coconut or jojoba oil)
- 1 drop sweet marjoram essential oil
- 1 drop clary sage essential oil
- 1 drop rose essential oil

Directions

Add the St John's wort oil (or light coconut or jojoba oil) to a glass or ceramic beaker or bowl. Add the essential oils one by one and stir with a glass rod to mix.

To use, massage onto the abdomen and lower back using a gentle clockwise motion. Use within 6 weeks, or within 12 months if made with coconut or jojoba oil.

ABDOMINAL RUB FOR CONSTIPATION

Constipation is best dealt with by combining herbal remedies with dietary changes and exercise. This recipe can help to alleviate some of the discomfort; the amount is enough for no more than a couple of applications, but you can also increase the proportions if you wish to make a larger batch if it is a recurrent issue. Grapeseed, apricot or sweet almond oil make good base oils, but for larger amounts, use light coconut or jojoba oil as these do not deteriorate with age.

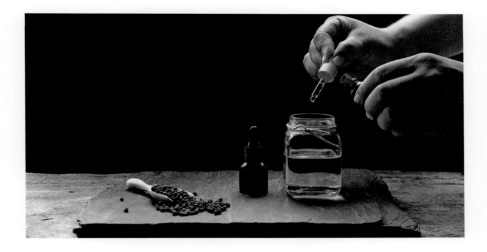

Ingredients

- 2 teaspoons grapeseed, apricot or sweet almond oil (or light coconut or jojoba oil)
- 1 drop black pepper essential oil
- 1 drop basil essential oil
- 1 drop cardamon essential oil

Directions

Add the carrier oil to a glass or ceramic beaker or bowl. Then add the essential oils one by one and stir with a glass rod to mix.

To use, massage onto the abdomen and lower back using a gentle clockwise motion. It is best used within 6 months, or one year if using coconut or jojoba oil.

TUMMY RUB FOR CRAMPS / IBS

Tummy cramps can be caused by several factors, including indigestion, wind and IBS as well being brought on by emotional distress. Our stomach is very sensitive and reacts quickly to emotional upsets even if we don't always recognize this connection. The recipe below is enough for no more than a couple of applications, but you can also increase the proportions if you wish to make a larger batch if it is a recurrent issue. Calendula oil is very soothing and healing, but for larger amounts, use light coconut or jojoba oil as they do not deteriorate with age.

Ingredients

- 2 teaspoons calendula oil (light coconut or jojoba oil)
- 1 drop fennel essential oil
- 1 drop peppermint essential oil
- 1 drop chamomile essential oil

Directions

Add the carrier oil to a glass or ceramic beaker or bowl. Add the essential oils one by one and stir with a glass rod to mix.

To use, massage onto the abdomen and lower back using a gentle clockwise motion.

It is best used within 6 months, or 12 months if using coconut or jojoba oil.

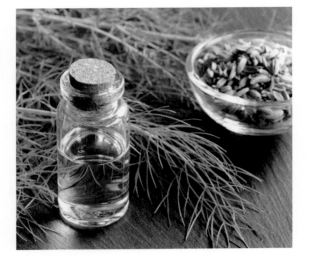

VARIATION

If you are making larger amounts, choose jojoba or coconut oil, which will keep well for over a year. Although very healing, calendula oil is best used within 6 months.

ARTHRITIS
+ JOINT BALM

This is an effective pain-relief balm for aching joints or arthritis. The recipe combines several healing infused oils with essential oils having analgesic and anti-inflammatory properties. Arthritis, rheumatism and all kinds of joint pain benefit from a multifaceted approach, which includes bathing in hot baths using salts and clays. It is best to apply this balm to joints when the skin is warm after bathing and to any areas of pain as often as required.

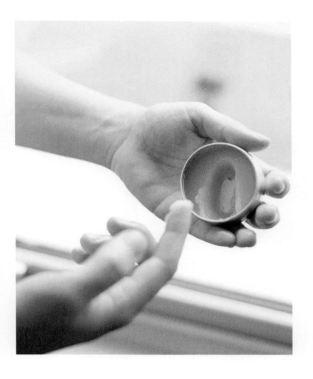

Ingredients

- 4 teaspoons calendula oil
- 1 tablespoon comfrey oil
- 1 tablespoon arnica oil
- 2 teaspoons St John's wort oil
- 2 teaspoons beeswax
- 8 drops rosemary essential oil
- 8 drops lavender essential oil
- 8 drops white thyme essential oil

Directions

Place a glass jug or bowl over a small saucepan of water to create a bain-marie or use a double boiler. Bring the water to the boil and then reduce to a simmer. Keep on the heat until everything has melted, stirring regularly with a spoon or glass rod.

Remove from the heat and add the essential oils one by one. Stir well.

Pour the balm mix into a glass jar or aluminium tin and allow the mix to set for approximately 20 minutes.

Once it has set, it is ready to use. Apply the balm directly to the joints after bathing.

COUGHS + COLDS CHEST BALM

This vapour rub is good for soothing coughing and as an expectorant to help ease congestion. The essential oils all have powerful bactericidal and antiviral actions, which help to combat infection. Rosemary is my favourite go-to remedy if you feel a cold or cough coming on as it will stop it from fully developing – in this case, it is good to use rosemary oil in rubs, baths, steam inhalations and in room diffusers to get the maximum effect.

Ingredients

- 60 ml (2 fl oz) grapeseed or light coconut oil
- 1 teaspoon shea butter
- 2 teaspoons beeswax
- 10 drops eucalyptus (or ravensara) essential oil
- 10 drops peppermint essential oil
- 10 drops rosemary essential oil
- 10 drops fragonia or tea tree essential oil

Directions

Place a glass jug or bowl over a small saucepan of water to create a bain-marie or use a double boiler. Add the grapeseed or coconut oil, shea butter and beeswax to the glass bowl. Bring the water to the boil and then reduce to a simmer.

Once liquified and warmed, remove from the heat and add the essential oils one by one. Stir with a glass rod to combine fully, then pour into a sterilized glass jar or container. Leave to set for 10 to 15 minutes.

To use, rub the ointment on the throat and chest areas.

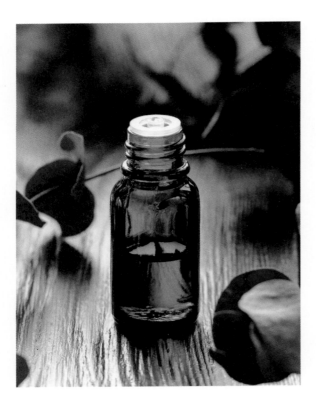

STEAM INHALATION FOR CONGESTION

Steam inhalation is an age-old method for easing congestion. Adding essential oils such as eucalyptus, tea tree, white thyme, ravensara or rosemary to the water helps to further clear the passageways in your nose and sinuses. These oils also all have bactericidal actions which help to kill germs and viruses and fight infection.

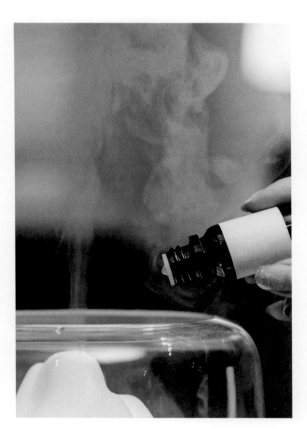

Ingredients

- 1.5 litres (50 fl oz; about 1 kettle-full) boiling water
- 1 drop white thyme essential oil
- 1 drop eucalyptus essential oil
- 1 drop rosemary essential oil

Directions

Pour the boiling water carefully into a bowl. Add the essential oils one by one.

Sit with your head over the bowl of hot water, placing a towel over your head and the bowl to collect the steam. Close your eyes and breathe deeply for up to 3 minutes. Avoid getting the hot steam in your eyes.

HAYFEVER REMEDY ROLLERBALL

Fragonia water and fragonia essential oil have been shown to provide relief from hay fever in some individuals, and are helpful for allergies or coughs.

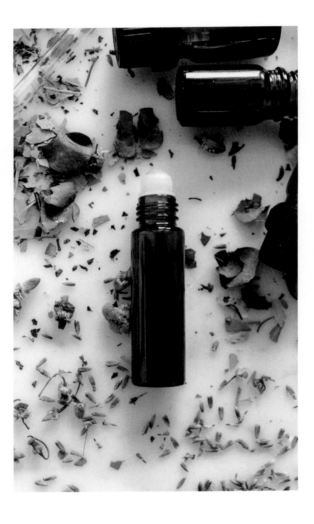

Ingredients

o   2 teaspoons calendula oil
o   3 drops sandalwood essential oil
o   7 drops fragonia essential oil
o   3 drops rosemary essential oil

Directions

Fill a 10-ml (⅓-fl oz) rollerball bottle with the carrier oil. Add the essential oils one by one. Put the roller ball lid and cap on tightly and shake well.

To use, apply a little of this oil blend under the nostrils and on pulse points several times a day for best results.

It is best to use rollerball blends based on infused oils within 6 weeks but those based on jojoba or coconut oil will last at least 12 months.

5+ Medicine

TRAVEL SICKNESS ROLLERBALL

This is a useful aid to help overcome any travel sickness issues on the go.

Ingredients

- 2 teaspoons light coconut or grapeseed oil
- 3 drops ginger essential oil
- 4 drops grapefruit essential oil
- 5 drops peppermint essential oil

Directions

Fill a 10-ml (⅓-fl oz) rollerball bottle with the carrier oil. Add the essential oils one by one. Put the roller ball lid and cap on and shake well.

To use, apply to pulse points liberally before and during travel or roll under your nose. Alterntatively dab on a tissue and inhale the scent.

MIDLIFE + MENOPAUSE ROLLERBALL

This remedial rollerball is easy to pop into your handbag for frequent use throughout the day, as needed.

Ingredients

- ½ teaspoon evening primrose oil
- ½ teaspoon St John's wort oil
- 1 teaspoon light coconut oil
- 3 drops clary sage essential oil
- 3 drops geranium essential oil
- 2 drops spearmint essential oil
- 2 drops lavender essential oil
- 2 drops bergamot essential oil

Directions

Fill a 10-ml (⅓-fl oz) rollerball bottle with the carrier oils. Add essential oils one by one. Put the roller ball lid and cap on and shake well.

To use, apply to pulse points liberally, massage into the soles of your feet or roll along your hands. Then take 10 deep expansive breaths to inhale the scent.

LIFESTYLE TIP

My essential travel kit includes lavender, rosemary, tea tree, peppermint and citronella essential oils, plus jojoba oil and fragonia (or neroli) flower water.

BITE RELIEF REMEDY ROLLERBALL

OIL PULLING FOR MOUTH + GUM HEALTH

This is an excellent first aid remedy, especially while travelling, as it provides relief from mosquitoes and other biting insects.

Ingredients

o   2 teaspoons calendula oil
o   5 drops chamomile essential oil
o   5 drops lavender essential oil
o   2 drops yarrow essential oil

Directions

Fill a 10-ml (⅓-fl oz) rollerball bottle with the carrier oil. Add essential oils one by one. Put the roller ball lid and cap on and shake well.

To use, apply liberally to bites, such as those from mosquitoes, several times a day for best results.

Oil pulling is an age-old ayurvedic remedy, known as *gundusha*, that uses vegetable oils to clean and detoxify the teeth and gums. It can also help to whiten the teeth and is very beneficial for gum health. Activated charcoal is also helpful in promoting the correct pH balance and preventing cavities, tooth decay and gingivitis. Oil pulling is best done in the morning, before eating or drinking anything, but it can also be done before each meal if needed, for more severe infections or dental problems.

Ingredients

o   1–2 teaspoons coconut, sesame or olive oil (ideally organic)
o   ½ teaspoon activated charcoal
o   ½ teaspoon sea salt
o   Warm water

Directions

Put 1–2 teaspoons of coconut oil into the mouth. Swish around your mouth for up to 20 minutes – the timing is key as this is long enough to break down plaque and bacteria but not long enough for the body to start re-absorbing any toxins. The oil will become thicker and milky as it mixes with saliva, and it will turn creamy white.

Spit out into the toilet – not the sink – to avoid any future blockages. Rinse well with a little activated charcoal mixed into warm, salty water.

CLOVE TOOTH + GUM REMEDY

Rinsing the mouth with warm water and salt is a traditional and effective remedy for sore, bleeding gums, toothache, mouth ulcers or abscesses. When this is combined with the powerful bactericidal and antiseptic actions of clove, it becomes even more effective. Just chewing on a clove bud can help numb the pain due to toothache — alternatively you can put one drop of clove essential oil on a cotton bud and apply to the painful tooth or abscess. This recipe can be used for all kinds of mouth or gum problems, including ulcers or abscesses.

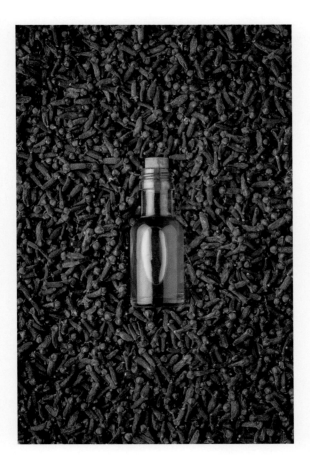

Ingredients

- 2 drops clove essential oil (or 3 clove buds)
- 1 teaspoon light coconut oil
- 1 teaspoon sea salt

Directions

Use 2 drops of clove oil; alternatively, crush the cloves in pestle and mortar and add to the coconut oil. Mix in a sprinkle of sea salt to create a paste.

To use, apply this to the sore area of the mouth or gums several times a day for relief.

VARIATION

Add clove essential oil to jojoba or coconut oil to use as a topical pain-relief remedy or to ease itching.

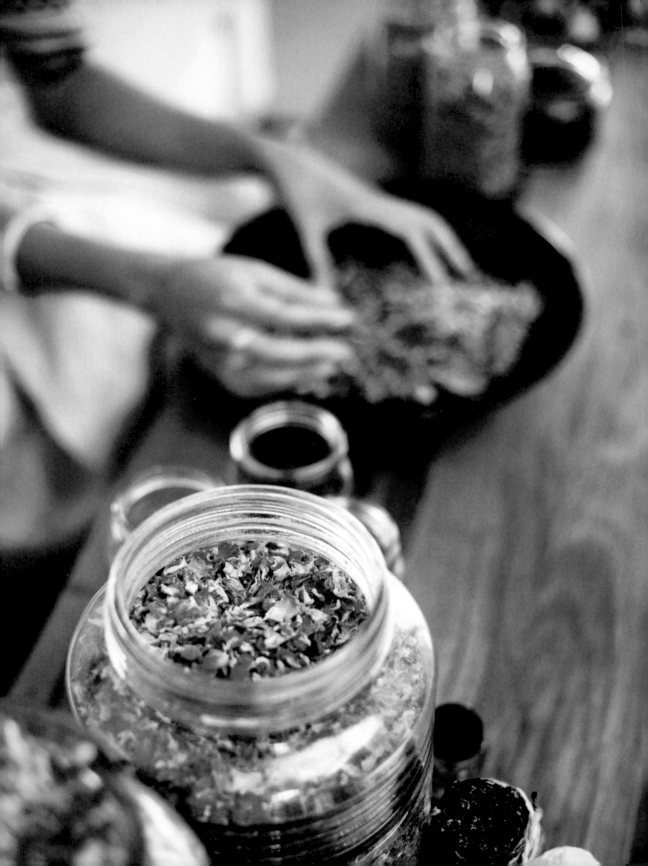

A GUIDE TO NATURAL

RAW MATERIALS

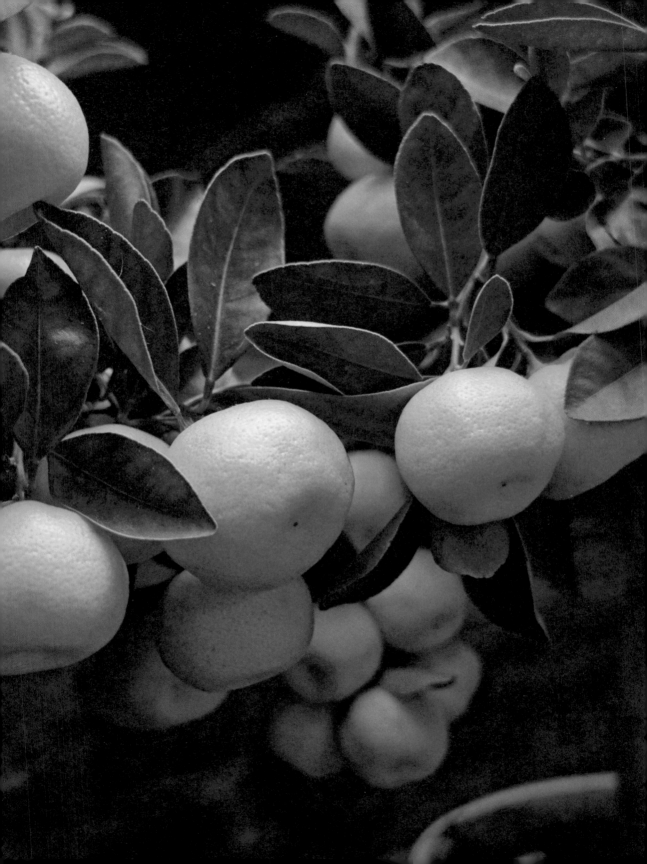

ESSENTIAL OILS

Essential oils are highly aromatic, volatile plant oils that are used in the practice of aromatherapy. These oils tend to evaporate easily at room temperature, and it is this volatile character that allows their aroma to be perceived as fragrant. All essential oils, such as peppermint, lavender and geranium, have a unique phytochemical composition that is responsible for the highly distinctive aroma of the plant.

Essential oils are extracted from the plant material in several ways: some are extracted by simply pressing the fresh plant, as in the case of orange peel oil; but in most cases essential oils are extracted by passing steam through the herb; delicate flowers are best prepared by the method of 'enfleurage'. In general, a great deal of plant material is necessary to extract even a small amount of the pure essential oils. Here is a selection of the most useful ones.

AGONIS FRAGRANS **FRAGONIA**	A pale oil with a slightly citrus, fresh, clean scent. It displays most of the medicinal characteristics of tea tree, being an excellent anti-infectious, bactericidal and fungicidal oil, yet it has a pleasing smell. It blends well with citrus oils.
BOSWELLIA CARTERI **FRANKINCENSE**	A warm, rich, sweet-balsamic oil with a sedating effect on the nervous system. It helps to calm the mind and is well known as an ingredient of incense in the East and West. It has a healing, rejuvenating effect on the skin. In blending, it makes a very useful base note, especially in combination with other resins such as elemi or myrrh.
CANANGA ODORATA VAR. GENUINA **YLANG YLANG**	An exquisite perfume oil, with a deep, soft, floral-balsamic fragrance. It has a marked sedating effect on the nerves but is reviving to the spirit – a traditional aphrodisiac! This oil is a well-balanced perfume in its own right but can also be used to add an exotic, rich and sensual element to blends.
CEDRUS ATLANTICA **CEDARWOOD ATLAS**	A woody-balsamic oil having a sedative effect on the nerves, traditionally burnt as an incense and used to repel insects. Good for skincare and respiratory complaints. It blends well with cypress, jasmine, juniper, clary sage, vetiver, rosemary and ylang ylang.

CHAMAEMELUM NOBILE **ROMAN CHAMOMILE**	Both Roman and German chamomile (*Matricaria recutita*) have a rich green-apple scent and share similar properties. They are both excellent sedative and antispasmodic oils, though German chamomile is a superior anti-inflammatory agent for skincare. They blend well with lavender, bergamot, clary sage, jasmine, neroli, rose and geranium.
CITRUS AURANTIFOLIA **LIME**	A fresh, sweet-fruity citrus scent that has an uplifting effect on the mind and a cleansing effect on the systems of the body. It is a very useful oil to use in blends to add a pleasingly sweet top note as it combines well with most other oils. **Note:** The expressed oil is phototoxic when applied to skin exposed to direct sunlight.
CITRUS AURANTIUM VAR. AMARA **NEROLI**	An intensely rich, floral perfume, reputed to have aphrodisiac properties. It is uplifting to the mind and spirit but soothing to the nervous system. It is a good skincare oil that blends well with benzoin, jasmine, myrrh, lavender, rose and all citrus oils.
CITRUS AURANTIUM VAR. AMARA **PETITGRAIN**	Extracted from the leaf, with a fresh, floral citrus scent, somewhat similar to neroli. A classic ingredient of eau-de-cologne, it gives a twist to an otherwise flat composition, having a unique quality as a top note in blends.
CITRUS SINENSIS **SWEET ORANGE**	A sweet, familiar, citrus-scented oil, which has a sedating effect on the digestion and nervous system. Adds warmth to any blends and combines well with lavender, clary sage, neroli, myrrh, frankincense and other citrus oils. **Note:** The distilled oil is phototoxic when applied to skin exposed to direct sunlight.
COMMIPHORA MYRRHA **MYRRH**	A rich, warming oil with a spicy-balsamic aroma, which has been used as a remedy for over 3,000 years! It has a marked healing, rejuvenating effect on the skin and, as such, it is a useful oil to include in skincare blends. It blends well with frankincense, benzoin, sandalwood, cypress, juniper, patchouli, lavender and spice oils.
CUPRESSUS SEMPERVIRENS **CYPRESS**	A sweet, smoky-balsamic fragrance. A good astringent with a sedative effect on the nervous system, traditionally used as an incense and for skincare – it also has good detox properties. It blends well with cedarwood, pine, lavender, juniper, orange, marjoram and sandalwood.

CYMBOPOGON CITRATUS **LEMONGRASS**	A fresh grassy-lemony scented oil, which has good anti-infectious properties and a sedative effect on the nervous system. It blends well with other citrus oils but can be quite overpowering in blends if not used in moderation.
CYMBOPOGON MARTINII **PALMAROSA**	A light green oil with a sweet, floral, rosy-green scent, good for all types of skin. A useful oil to provide the heart of a blend as a middle note as it 'rounds off' other scents. It blends especially well with citrus oils
CYMBOPOGON NARDUS **CITRONELLA**	A powerful, fresh, lemony-scented oil. It has a stimulating effect on the nervous system and is traditionally used to repel mosquitoes. It blends well with geranium, pine, cypress and other citrus oils.
EUCALYPTUS GLOBULUS **EUCALYPTUS**	A clear, camphoraceous oil with a strong, penetrating, stimulating odour, well known for its decongestant properties and as a powerful anti-infectious oil. It blends well with rosemary, lavender, clary sage, marjoram and herbal oils.
FOENICULUM VULGARE **SWEET FENNEL**	A sweet, anise-like scented oil, it has a cleansing effect on the systems of the body, and is good for cellulite reduction and to detox. It blends well with geranium, lavender, rose, chamomile and sandalwood.
JASMINUM OFFICINALE **JASMINE**	An exquisite perfume oil, with an intense floral fragrance. It has an uplifting, soothing quality though it has a stimulating effect on the nervous system. An aphrodisiac and a good skincare oil, it blends well with other florals such as neroli and rose, and also has the quality of 'rounding off' just about any blend.
JUNIPERUS COMMUNIS **JUNIPER**	A fresh, woody-balsamic oil, traditionally used as a blood cleanser, it has a purifying effect on the systems of the body. It blends well with vetiver, sandalwood, cedarwood, clary sage, geranium, benzoin and citrus oils. **Note:** Contra-indicated for those with kidney problems.
LAVANDULA ANGUSTIFOLIA **LAVENDER**	A familiar oil with a sweet, floral fragrance and a multitude of uses! It has a marked sedating effect on the nervous system and makes a multipurpose healing skincare remedy. It also blends well with most oils so is therefore perhaps the most useful oil to keep in any blending kit.

MELALEUCA ALTERNIFOLIA
TEA TREE

A very useful medicinal oil with a fresh, camphoraceous, powerful odour. It supports the immune system and is active against bacteria, fungi and viruses. It blends well with other medicinal or herbal oils, such as rosemary, peppermint and ravensara. **Note:** May cause sensitization in some individuals.

MENTHA PIPERITA
PEPPERMINT

This penetrating, minty oil is cooling and refreshing – it clears the head and revives the spirit. A good travel companion – especially for respiratory and digestive problems of a nervous origin. It blends well with rosemary and other refreshing herbal oils.

MYRTUS COMMUNIS
MYRTLE

This fresh-smelling essential oil inhibits infection, since it is a bactericidal, germicidal, fungicidal and antiviral agent – in this respect it has some similarities to tea tree oil. It is effective against many types of respiratory infections and, used in a room vaporizer, it helps clears congestion resulting from airborne infections; it also supports the immune system and nervous system. It blends well with lavender, rosemary, clary sage, bay, lime, clove and other spice oils.

OCIMUM BASILICUM
SWEET BASIL

This oil has a sweet-herbaceous scent. It has a refreshing, clearing and purifying effect on the mind and a stimulating and fortifying effect on the body. It blends well with clary sage, bergamot, lime, marjoram, lavender and geranium.

ORIGANUM MAJORANA
SWEET MARJORAM

A warm, nutty aroma, which has a strong sedating effect on the mind and the nervous system, and a powerful anti-spasmodic action on the muscles of the body. It blends well with lavender, rosemary, bergamot, chamomile, cedarwood and cypress.

PELARGONIUM GRAVEOLENS
GERANIUM

A sweet, rosy-green scented oil, which has a balancing and harmonizing effect on the nervous system. It is an excellent all-purpose oil for skincare and makes a valuable middle note in blending work, as it combines well with most oils.

PIMENTA RACEMOSA
BAY

This oil has fresh spicy top note and sweet-balsamic undertone. It promotes hair growth and can help combat dandruff. Extensively used in fragrances, especially for men, it blends well with lavender, geranium, ylang yang and spice oils.

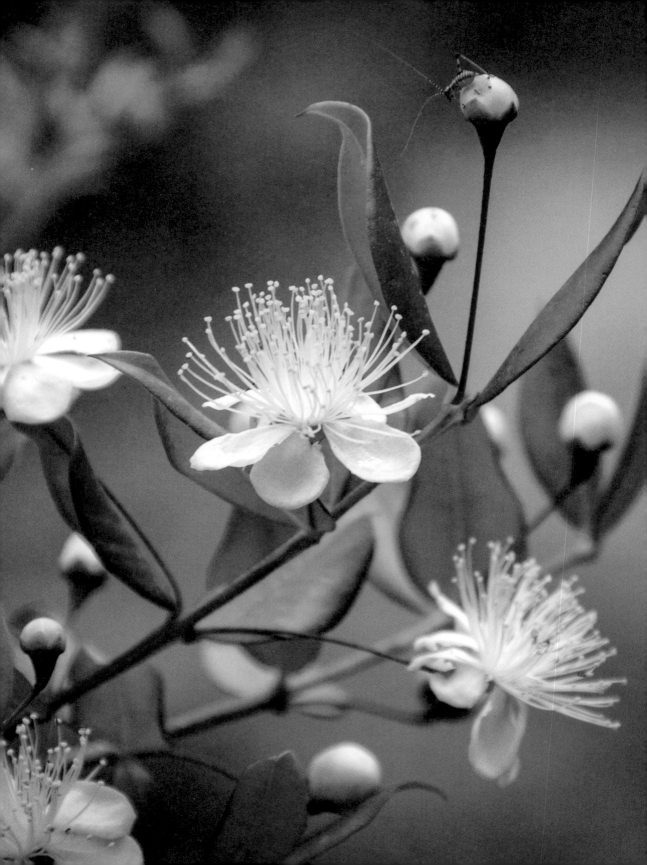

PINUS SYLVESTRIS
PINE

This fresh, balsamic scented oil is a useful antiseptic, with a stimulating and refreshing effect, and good for respiratory problems. It blends well with other woody and spicy oils.

PIPER NIGRUM
BLACK PEPPER

One of the most ancient spices, which has been in use for over 4,000 years. The pungent, light amber oil has a warming and stimulating effect on the whole system and helps fortify the muscles. It blends well with most oils when used in small amounts.

POGOSTEMON CABLIN
PATCHOULI

This rich, musky-earthy oil has strong associations with the East, where it is used to scent cloth. It soothes the mind, supports the nervous system and is a potent aphrodisiac. May be used a perfume on its own or combined with other exotic oils.

RAVENSARA AROMATICA
RAVENSARA

This oil has a fresh, slightly lemony, slightly camphoraceous scent and has powerful antiviral, antifungal and bactericidal properties. Valuable for combatting respiratory and airborne infections, it also supports the nervous and immune systems. It blends well with rosemary, eucalyptus, tea tree, fragonia, bay and spice oils.

ROSA CENTIFOLIA
ROSE MAROC

This beautiful, feminine scent has long been associated with love. It warms the heart and soothes the nerves. It is especially suitable for children and those with sensitive skin. It is also one of the most useful skincare oils because it helps in the daily process of skin repair and keeps the skin lubricated and elastic, making it less prone to wrinkles. Suited to all types of complexion, particularly dry, sensitive and ageing or mature skin, it blends well with virtually everything!

SALVIA ROSMARINUS
ROSEMARY

A penetrating oil with a warm, herbal fragrance and strong stimulating and fortifying properties. In blends, it is one of the most useful medicinally active ingredients and combines well with most other herbal oils, such as clary sage, marjoram and lavender. **Note:** Contraindicated for those with high blood pressure and epileptics.

SALVIA SCLAREA
CLARY SAGE

A pleasing, sweet, nutty-herbaceous scent. It is especially good for stress and anxiety states, in comparison to Spanish sage (*Salvia lavandulifolia*), which is more stimulating. It blends well with juniper, lavender, geranium, sandalwood, cedarwood, frankincense, bergamot and other herbal oils. **Note:** Clary sage oil should not be used in combination with drinking alcohol.

**SANTALUM
ALBUM
SANDALWOOD**

This incense, cosmetic and perfume material has enjoyed over 4,000 years of uninterrupted use. The oil has a deep, soft, woody-balsamic scent, which is soothing and very long- lasting. It is a well-known aphrodisiac and useful skincare remedy and combines well with lavender, black pepper, bergamot, patchouli, myrrh and jasmine.

**STYRAX
BENZOIN
BENZOIN**

A resinous, rich essential oil with a sweet, vanilla-like aroma. It has a comforting and soothing effect on the heart and emotions; a cleansing and energizing effect on the systems of the body. A good skincare oil, which blends well with rose, sandalwood, frankincense, jasmine, myrrh, cypress, juniper and spice oils.

**SYZYGIUM
AROMATICUM
CLOVE**

The oil has a warm, strong, spicy smell that is stimulating to the mind, helping lift depression and ease respiratory problems. Invaluable for mouth, gum and tooth infections and pain. It masks unpleasant odours and repels insects. The oil is useful to add a warm, spicy element to blends when added in small amounts.

**THYMUS
VULGARIS
WHITE THYME**

There are numerous varieties of thyme, but of these the 'white' thyme oil is recommended for aromatherapy and home use. It has a herby, fresh-green scent and is valuable for circulatory, respiratory and nervous complaints. It blends well with other herbaceous oils, including rosemary, lavender, marjoram and clary sage.

**VETIVERIA
ZIZANIOIDES
VETIVER**

A very soothing and relaxing oil with a soft, earthy undertone and a sweet woody top note, known in the East as 'the oil of tranquillity'. It blends well with patchouli, rose, sandalwood, lavender, ylang ylang and clary sage.

**ZINGIBER
OFFICINALE
GINGER**

The oil has a warm, spicy-woody aroma with a strong stimulating and warming effect on the entire system. Valuable used in small amounts in blends to add a hint of warmth and body to a blend.

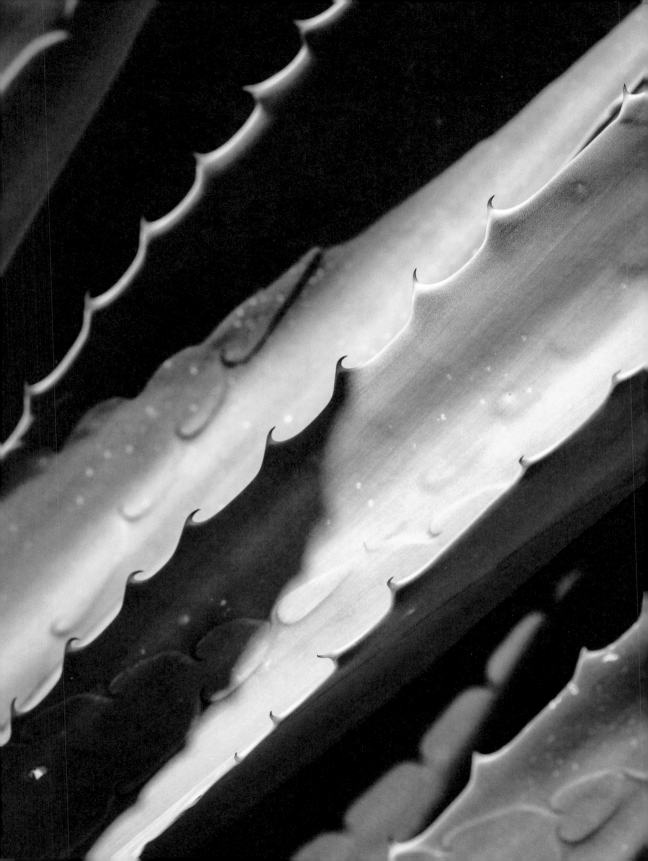

VEGETABLE OILS, WAXES + BUTTERS

Vegetable oils or 'carrier' oils are generally produced by compression, from the seeds, nuts, fruit or kernels of a plant, such as sweet almond oil (kernel), grape seed oil (seed), coconut oil (nut) or olive oil (fruit). In the case of avocado, the thick oil is made from the actual pulp of the fruit, which is full of natural, healthy unsaturated fats. Jojoba oil is actually a liquid wax while raw coconut oil is solid at room temperature and acts more like a butter. Cold-pressed, organically produced oils and butters are of the highest quality since they retain all their nutritional value.

ALOE BARBADENSIS
ALOE VERA BUTTER

A fantastic moisturizer with a silky-soft feel. The anti-inflammatory aloe vera butter also naturally contains lignin, which helps to draw other recipe ingredients into the deeper layers of the skin.

ARGANIA SPINOSA
ARGAN OIL

Renowned for its skin moisturizing and repairing properties. It is very rich in antioxidants, vitamin E, squalene, phytosterols and essential fatty acids so it is a perfect oil to use in a facial serum for reducing fine lines and wrinkles. Argan is also a natural anti-inflammatory and helps to balance sebum production in oily skins, reducing acne. Used in body oils, it increases elasticity, leaving the skin feeling firmer with an overall smoother appearance. Argan is also beneficial for promoting hair health and growth, leaving it silky, shiny and soft.

BORAGO OFFICINALIS
BORAGE OIL

Also called starflower, this has the highest concentration of the essential fatty acid omega-6 as well as gamma-linolenic acid (GLA), making it the richest plant source of essential fatty acids! As such, it can be used as an anti-ageing treatment all on its own or can be added to oils or serums for its rejuvenating effect. It also quickly restores moisture and elasticity to dry or sun-damaged skin as well having a healing effect on skin disorders such as eczema and dermatitis.

**BUXUS
CHINENSIS
JOJOBA OIL**

Actually a liquid wax rather than an oil: the terms jojoba 'oil' and jojoba 'wax' are often used interchangeably because the wax visually appears to be like a mobile oil. It is a very valuable healing substance, especially for skincare, where its unique composition accounts for its amazing shelf-life stability compared with many of the 'true' vegetable oils. It also displays an extraordinary resistance to high temperatures. It has no smell and does not go rancid, so it makes an ideal base for body lotions or facial oils. A fantastic hair and skin conditioner, jojoba is very similar in consistency to the sebum in our skin, so is one of nature's best natural moisturizers: perfect for mature, dry, ageing and sensitive skin. It is also anti-inflammatory, good for oily or acne-prone skin. Jojoba wax also makes a good alternative ingredient to beeswax for use by vegans.

**CALENDULA
ARVENSIS
CALENDULA
OIL**

Rich in vitamins C and E, the plant has been used for centuries to heal a range of skin complaints, including wounds, blemishes, burns, eczema, inflammations and bruises. Calendula also has proven antifungal and antiseptic properties.

**CAMELLIA
OLEIFERA
CAMELLIA
SEED OIL**

From the seeds of the white tea plant, camellia is a traditional cosmetic oil used for centuries in China and Japan. Lightweight and faintly aromatic, it has a silk-like feel that sinks easily into the skin without leaving an oily finish. It has exceptional moisturizing, rejuvenating and antioxidant qualities, being abundant in anti-ageing nutrients including oleic acids, linoleic acids, squalene, vitamins A, B and E and beneficial minerals, including phosphorus, calcium, iron, manganese and magnesium.

**COCOS
NUCIFERA
COCONUT OIL**

A fantastic moisturizer, rich in natural fats plus squalene and vitamin E. Traditionally used to nourish and moisturize both skin and hair, it makes a versatile conditioning agent. Coconut oil also has natural antibacterial properties, making it valuable for oily skin and acne. 'Light' coconut oil, which is absorbed more easily and quickly, is a good make-up remover / facial cleanser. Light coconut oil is a very stable material that does not deteriorate with age, making it a perfect base for massage oils, perfumes and facial oils.

**CORYLUS
AVELLANA
HAZELNUT OIL**

Rich in oleic acid, a fatty acid that helps to moisturize the skin and keep it hydrated. It is known for its hydrating properties, as it is high in vitamin E and fatty acids, which can help in keeping the skin soft and supple. Hazelnut oil also boosts collagen production and has anti-ageing effects by reducing wrinkles and the appearance of scars and dark spots caused by hyperpigmentation. It is one of the best oils for oily or acne-prone skin, as it is antibacterial and acts like an astringent, which helps prevent excess oil production. With the presence of linoleic acid, it also nourishes hair follicles to promote healthier and stronger hair growth and can alleviate dry scalps and restore dry and brittle ends.

DUNALIELLA SALINA CARROT OIL

A unique unicellular species of algae harvested from the Dead Sea and containing rich concentrations of carotenoids (mainly betacarotene), antioxidants and essential vitamins. Extracted from a sea algae found in salt fields, it is then produced for use in a base oil. With powerful antioxidant properties, this valuable oil helps skin resist the damaging effects of the sun and premature ageing, including sunspots. Use in regenerative skincare, as it stimulates skin cell growth and maintains the elasticity of skin. This oil can be applied to the skin direct or blended with essential oils for an aromatic massage. It also reinforces the immune system and slows down ageing and cell degradation. **Note:** It is not extracted from carrots, despite the common name, and should not be confused with carrot seed essential oil!

HIPPOPHAE RHAMNOIDES SEA BUCKTHORN OIL

An abundant source of many nutrients and minerals, with six different vitamins, 22 fatty acids and 42 kinds of lipids, which makes it an excellent choice for any skin in need of hydration or nutrition.

HYPERICUM PERFORATUM ST JOHN'S WORT OIL

A dark red infused oil with a strong odour, traditionally used as wound-healing salve. Key benefits include its antiviral, antibacterial and antioxidant properties, which are good for inflamed or damaged skin and sunburn, and also to soothe damaged nerves. It is used for the treatment of minor wounds and burns, sunburn, abrasions and bruises. In skincare, it moisturizes dry skin and helps to heal pimples, eczema, dermatitis and psoriasis – the active ingredients in the oil soothe the skin and relieve itching.

LIMNANTHES ALBA MEADOWFOAM SEED OIL

Composed of mostly fatty acids and antioxidants, having a lightweight, non-oily texture. It is absorbed easily into the skin and does not feel heavy or greasy, so is suitable for all skin types. It helps fight free-radical damage to dehydrated skin, which is one of the main causes of wrinkles, and it can also help to reduce the appearance of fine lines or sunspots.

**MACADAMIA
INTEGRIFOLIA
MACADAMIA
OIL**

Produced from the nuts of a tree native to Australia, macadamia oil is deeply emollient and a rich source of omegas. The palmitoleic acid and squalene present in the oil helps to prevent the premature formation of wrinkles by boosting the regeneration of skin keratinocytes. Linoleic acid also helps to reduce trans-epidermal water loss, keeping the skin well hydrated and supple – the oil is also rich in fatty acids and potassium. This oil is a perfect conditioner for all hair types, especially beneficial to dry, damaged hair.

**OENOTHERA
BIENNIS
EVENING
PRIMROSE OIL**

Rich in vitamins, minerals and essential fatty acids, including gamma-linolenic acid (GLA). Our body converts the GLA in the evening primrose oil into hormone-like substances called prostaglandins, which offer anti-inflammatory benefits and help to regulate hormones. GLA is also essential for cell structure, nerve function and the elasticity of the skin. The oil is great for hormonal skin while hydrating and moisturizing and improving skin's elasticity. It is especially good for dry or mature skin and eczema.

**ORYZA SATIVA
RICE BRAN OIL**

Used extensively in Japan to protect and soothe the skin, the oil is rich in natural plant sterols and the antioxidant gamma oryzanol and has anti-inflammatory properties. Very high in vitamin E, which helps to boost the protective quality of the skin cells and is directly connected to the health and wellness of the skin, including the healing of wounds, increasing cellular regeneration, reducing wrinkles and providing some protection from sunburn.

**PERSEA
GRATISSIMA
AVOCADO OIL**

Very rich in nutrients, which despite its thick consistency it delivers deep into the skin: these include vitamins A, D, B1, B2 pantothenic acid, E, lecithin and essential fatty acids. Sun- damaged skin and mature complexions especially benefit from avocado oil, and it can help protect against ultraviolet rays – it is also superb as a hair conditioner.

**PRUNUS
ARMENIACA
APRICOT
KERNEL OIL**

A light oil rich in vitamins A, D and E plus oleic and linoleic acids. It is non-greasy and is easily absorbed by the skin – ideal as a moisturizing and conditioning oil for mature and sensitive as well as inflamed or dry skin. Suitable for babies.

**PRUNUS DULCIS
SWEET ALMOND
OIL**

Moisturizing and nourishing, it makes an ideal massage oil base, leaving the skin soft and smooth without feeling greasy. It is rich in essential fatty acids as well as vitamins A, B1, B2, B6 and E. It is used for dry, itchy skin and as a hair treatment, and makes an excellent serum, especially for oily skins due to its lack of greasiness, and as a cuticle oil.

PRUNUS PERSICA
PEACH KERNEL OIL

A fine-textured, golden oil with a delicate, sweet aroma. It contains minerals and vitamins, especially vitamin E. An excellent moisturizing agent, high in fatty acids and antioxidant vitamins, it can be applied to the skin direct or blended with essential oils for an aromatic massage. Ideal for facial massage, especially for dry, ageing or sensitive skin and thread veins. Also suitable for children and babies.

ROSA RUBIGINOSA
ROSEHIP SEED OIL

Rich in retinoic acid found in vitamin A, which can help eliminate fine lines and wrinkles, the powerful antioxidants and omega fatty acids also protect cells from premature ageing. Best used in facial serums for sunspots or acne scars – also in body oils to treat existing scars, stretch marks or blemishes.

THEOBROMA CACAO
COCOA BUTTER

A rich, moisturizing cream extracted from roasted cacao beans, the name means 'food of the gods' in ancient Greek. Pure cocoa butter is high in fatty acids, which deeply hydrate and nourish the skin while improving elasticity and tone. It forms a protective barrier that holds in moisture, so makes a wonderful addition to moisturizers, body lotions and lip balms.

TRITICUM VULGARE
WHEATGERM OIL

Loaded with vitamins and minerals, including vitamin E, which helps improve skin elasticity, while nourishing and moisturizing skin cells. Adding 5 per cent of wheatgerm oil to a body or facial oil acts as natural preservative, lengthening the life of the blend, plus adding nutrients.

VITAMIN E
VITAMIN E OIL

Extracted from natural plant oils such as wheatgerm or sunflower. Beware of a common synthetic substitute, called tocopheryl acetate, so check the label first. The pure oil is both a nutrient and antioxidant and is extremely versatile. It helps neutralize free radicals, which damage skin cells, and it is also known for its anti-ageing and healing properties, valuable for treating mature skin, scars and stretch marks. Adding 5 per cent of pure vitamin E oil to a blend also acts as natural preservative and will lengthen its shelf life.

VITELLARIA PARADOXA
SHEA BUTTER

Extracted from the plant seeds, it contains high concentrations of fatty acids and vitamins and also has anti-inflammatory and healing properties. Using shea butter on the body, especially the face, can soften, tone and soothe the skin.

VITIS VINIFERA
GRAPESEED OIL

Light and easily absorbed, making it a useful a non-greasy, body oil ingredient, grapeseed oil is a rich source of linoleic acid (omega 6), which is important for protecting skin cell membranes. It is also good used as a hair conditioner.

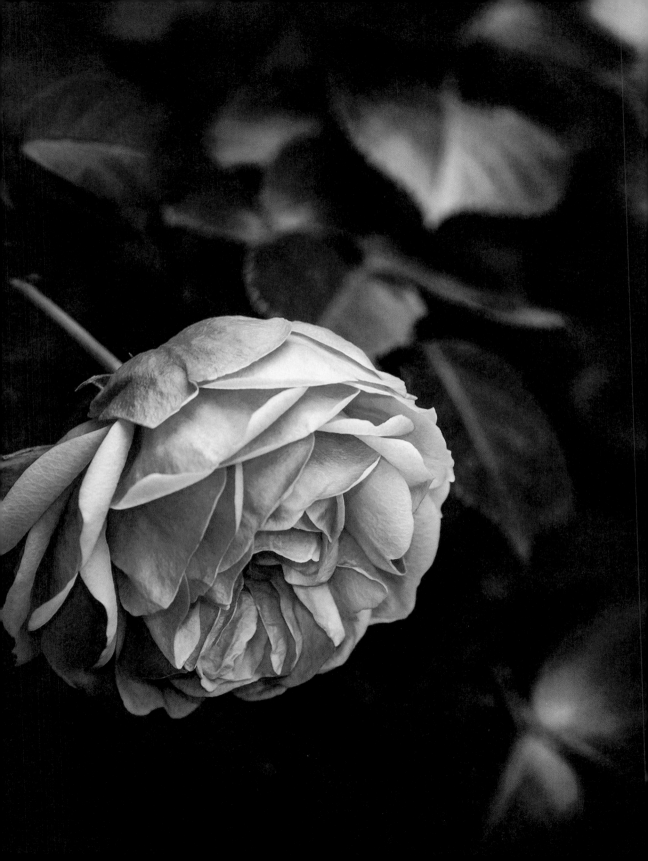

FLOWER WATERS

Water is essential to life! Pure water is vital for the effective functioning of our body with approximately 70 per cent of our body mass being made up of it. Since we lose water in large quantities every day, we need to replace it continually. But we use water not just to quench our thirst or for our personal hygiene, water has also been used therapeutically for centuries for cleansing and purifying our skin, cosmetically and via bathing. Today we can buy a range of spring waters from different sources that have healing qualities due to their specific combination of minerals. All our Aqua Oleum flower waters are made using spring water, rather than purified water, so they contain these healing and beneficial minerals. Commercially purified water which has been stripped of all its mineral content, can leach beneficial minerals out of our skin when applied locally, so it should be avoided. Micellar water has become fashionable in recent years as a quick cleanser, but this is made up of micelles (tiny balls) of cleansing molecules suspended in soft water: fundamentally, it is a mixture of soap and water. However, the ingredients used in micellar water leave a surface residue on the skin that can create a slight film, blocking the pores and disrupting the natural oil secretions of the skin. Floral waters are 100 per cent natural and all have specific therapeutic properties, being suitable even for the most sensitive skin. Use them as toners or for lightly cleansing the skin, or, if you prefer, just as a refreshingly fragrant spritz!

CITRONELLA WATER

This delightfully fresh flower water with an uplifting, lemony fragrance is suitable for use on the face and body. A safe and gentle bactericidal skin disinfectant, it makes the perfect toner / cleanser, especially for blemished or infected skin conditions. As a pick-me-up body freshener, it is reviving, stimulating as well as purifying. As an effective and proven natural mosquitos' repellent and protection, it can be applied to the face and body directly. Re-apply to exposed skin every few hours to provide protection from mosquitos.

FRAGONIA WATER

Completely unique to Aqua Oleum, fragonia water is especially good for those with acne, oily or blemished skin and for those who have skin prone to a sporadic flare-up of spots, as it has a purifying and antiseptic effect on the skin. In first aid, fragonia water is good for cleaning and disinfecting everyday cuts, bites or stings. The floral water also makes a lovely room freshener, having an uplifting, revitalizing and antidepressant effect. It is especially valuable to boost and support the immune system and to help prevent the spread of viral airborne infections within the home or office; in some individuals it can even help with bouts of asthma or hay fever. In addition, the spray makes a fantastic natural and fresh-smelling disinfectant for use around the home, when doing the laundry or for cleaning and wiping down surfaces. It makes a brilliant yoga mat spray!

GERANIUM **WATER**

This lovely, fragrant flower water can be used to help rebalance skin and the entire system in times of stress. Use it as a toner / cleanser in your daily skin routine, as it is especially ideal for combination skin, as well as for oily or blemished skin. As a cooling spritz, it can help soothe heat rash or menopausal flushes. Wear it as a natural perfume or use it as a light and fragrant air freshener in the summer; it is an all-time favourite with children. Don't forget to pack a bottle of geranium water in your carry-on when you travel to keep you feeling refreshed, your skin hydrated, and to help combat jet lag and travel sickness.

JASMINE **WATER**

Known in India as 'the perfume of love', this exquisite fragrant water has a sensual and exotic allure. The lovely floral scent is simultaneously revitalizing and energizing yet also calming and relaxing – ideal as a light perfume or fragrant body spritz. Studies suggest that it may even have a mild hypnotic or euphoric effect, making it valuable for anxiety, depression and stress-related conditions. Jasmine water makes a safe and gentle facial toner, particularly recommended for normal, dry and sensitive skin.

LAVENDER **WATER**

An all-time favourite, lavender aqua mist is a well-known relaxing remedy with a familiar, soothing floral fragrance. Lavender water can help soothe anxiety or agitation and it also works for children! Suitable for all skin types, especially blemished or acne-prone skin, it is best used as a gentle facial toner as part of a daily skin routine. It can also be used to clean minor cuts and grazes and to soothe insect bites or sunburned skin due to its healing properties, also making it an excellent travel companion. Spray it on your pillow to encourage a restful night's sleep.

MELISSA
WATER

Traditionally known as the 'elixir of life', melissa or lemon balm is renowned for its ability of help alleviate anxiety, depression, nervous tension, grief, heartache and all types of stress-related complaints. Simply inhaling this lemony-sweet, uplifting floral water helps to promote an overall feeling of calm and equilibrium, making it the perfect light perfume or body spritz. Remember to carry it with you whenever you feel you need a 'lift', as it provides an excellent way to freshen up naturally in dry conditions, hot weather and centrally heated rooms. Suitable for all skin types, especially sensitive and eczema-prone skin, as part of a daily skincare routine.

NEROLI
WATER

This is a personal favourite of mine. Neroli or orange blossom water has a delightful, fresh-green, soft fragrance, which is both refreshing and uplifting. As a rejuvenating and revitalizing facial tonic, it is especially suited to dry and sensitive skin. It also helps ease depression and anxiety when used as a light perfume or body spritz. Keep neroli water in your handbag when you are out and about, as this lovely, perfumed mist has a remarkable ability to reduce stress and calm anxiety while on the go!

ROSE
WATER

The most popular flower water and a quintessentially feminine, soothing lotion, rose water has been used for over 3,000 years! It has a multitude of skincare applications, being especially good for the care of mature and dry complexions. It also purifies the skin, tightens capillaries, reduces redness and closes the pores. Suitable for all skin types, it is best applied morning and night to cleanse and tone the skin. It's soft, floral and comforting scent is also deeply relaxing and an antidepressant with a soothing effect on the mind, making it an ideal on-the-go 'handbag' companion to keep you composed at all times, especially during the summer months.

ROSEMARY
WATER

This reviving flower water with a fresh-herbaceous fragrance makes the best all-round, uplifting morning pick-me-up spray for face and body. As a gently stimulating facial tonic, rosemary water can be used as an effective part of your daily skin routine; it is ideal for normal to oily skin. It can also help to reduce dark circles or puffiness beneath the eyes; plus, it increases blood flow to the skin. Spray directly on to damp hair as an excellent hair conditioner to encourage growth and impart shine. Keep a bottle in the fridge overnight for an especially invigorating and cooling 'hangover cure' facial spritz!

SPEARMINT
WATER

This herb has a long history for use to help relieve tension headaches and nausea as well as being good for fatigue, travel sickness and jet lag. It is also good applied as an light antiperspirant since menthol, the naturally occurring alcohol compound found in mint plants, causes a cooling, deodorant effect on the skin – lovely when used for refreshing tired feet after a long walk! A spearmint aqua spritz is a great go-to natural travel companion, especially for tropical climates or hot weather trips closer to home. It can be used as a toner in your daily skin routine, being ideal for oily, blemished and acne-prone skin. Try spraying a little on to the roots of your hair after it is towel dry to impart a soft fragrance and re-energize your scalp: its antiseptic and fungicidal properties can also help to reduce dandruff. In the home, use spearmint water to clean countertops and surfaces, as well as to repel mosquitos and ants.

TEA TREE
WATER

With outstanding antibacterial, antiseptic and antifungal properties, it makes a valuable addition to your first aid kit at home or abroad. This handy spray can be applied directly to soothe and clean insect bites, grazes, cuts and rashes, including sunburn. In skincare, it is ideal for treating oily, blemished and acne-prone complexions, and can be applied directly. It also makes an excellent antiseptic spray to help prevent the spread of viruses or airborne infections and can be employed as a natural household disinfectant; plus, it makes the perfect antiviral yoga mat spray!

WITCH HAZEL
WATER

A clear, colourless pure distillate with a fresh herbal-green fragrance, prepared from recently cut and partially dried twigs of *Hamamelis virginiana* containing natural oils and pure ethyl alcohol. This light aqua spray makes the perfect skin toner, which is especially beneficial for oily and blemished skin conditions. Naturally healing and bactericidal with outstanding astringent properties, it helps cleanse the skin of spots, blackheads and pimples while closing the pores. Popular as a yoga mat disinfectant spray in wellness studios, the flower water can also be used as the base for your own bactericidal spray. **Note:** Avoid contact with the eyes.

CLAYS

Clay comes in different consistencies where the specific colour of a clay derives from its unique mineral composition depending on the source of its extraction. The mineral composition gives each clay a specific action and, depending on your skin type and condition, one type of clay will work better for you than another. All clays draw oil from the skin, though some have stronger abilities than others. For instance, white clay is preferable for those who tend to have drier skin. Those with oilier skin, on the other hand, might choose Fuller's earth, which has super-absorbent properties. Cosmetic clays are commonly used in facial masks – combined with a flower water – and can be added to the bath for a mineral-infused soak or incorporated into dry shampoos.

BENTONITE CLAY

Composed of volcanic ash sediments that have been weathered over a long period of time, it is strongly absorbent, acting like a sponge when mixed with water. It has a mineral composition composed of mainly silica with iron, magnesium, calcium and potassium, plus other trace elements. Its high content of silica stimulates the production of protein and collagen, which explains its wide use for anti-ageing treatments – toning and restoring elasticity to demineralized and dull skin. It is great for rejuvenating and healing damaged tissue and for strengthening the hair and nails. Bentonite clay deeply cleans the scalp, removing dead skin cells and toxins – ideal for fine / oily hair – it also strengthens the hair and prevents hair loss by deep cleaning the hair follicles. Its high absorption properties remove grease and help tighten the skin, reducing the look of prominent pores. Suitable for all types of skin, bentonite clay is well suited for face, hair and scalp masks, foot baths, body packs, as well as for adding to baths.

FRENCH GREEN CLAY

With a mineral composition composed of mainly silica (45 per cent) with aluminium, iron, calcium, potassium, magnesium and phosphorus, plus trace elements, it has a light green tone when dry, with a rich green colour when hydrated – its verdant colour comes from decomposed plant matter within the clay. Green clay comes from the rich volcanic soils originally from France where it is famous for its healing action, deep detoxification and purification properties. Suitable for normal to oily skin and scalp, its therapeutic and beauty applications include face and hair masks, body wraps and clay baths.

FULLER'S EARTH CLAY

As this has strong oil-absorbent abilities, it is recommended for those with very oily skin. It also has mild natural bleaching properties. The dry clay has a lightly earthy scent and an off-white to greenish and tan colour. The texture is fine and powdery, so is very smooth and easy to mix with liquids. Suitable for normal to oily skin and scalp, the therapeutic and beauty applications include face and hair masks, body wraps and clay baths.

KAOLIN / WHITE CLAY

With a mineral composition of silica, calcium, magnesium, iron, potassium, aluminium and sodium, plus trace elements, white clay has a neutral pH for the skin, so it is recommended for all types of skin and scalp. The texture of the clay is very fine and soft and it has a gentle natural whitening action on the skin when used in facials and body treatments. In China, white kaolin clay is commonly used in porcelain and pottery. It's also found as an ingredient in toothpastes, cosmetics, skin- and haircare, and is a popular ingredient in many of the face masks on the market. It is not as absorbent as other clays, making it appropriate for skin that tends to be drier or more delicate. Because it has a pH value similar to the skin, white clay is especially suited to sensitive skin as well as for use as a natural baby powder – an ideal substitute to talc along with colloidal oatmeal. Use it in face, hair and scalp masks, body packs, clay baths and for personal hygiene.

RHASSOUL CLAY

A fine, red clay from Morocco that has been used for centuries in skincare, rhassoul is much gentler than many other clays and is typically recommended for more sensitive or mature skin types. It has a mineral composition composed of mainly silica, with potassium, iron and trace amounts of phosphorus, magnesium and calcium. This clay is rejuvenating and helps restore a youthful-looking complexion – especially suited to dry, mature and sensitive skin. It gently stimulates blood circulation – use it in face packs, hair masks, body wraps and baths. **Note:** Red clay can leave pigment on the surface of some types of skin after using as a facial or body mask. This is simply a concentration of red pigments which will later be absorbed.

SALTS

Salts and minerals are essential for our body to function! Salts can be used in different ways therapeutically in body scrubs and bath treatments as well as cosmetically. Different salts have specific properties depending on their composition and source. The soothing warmth and the natural buoyancy of bathing in warm water when salts are added to a hot bath contribute to their overall healing effect when they are absorbed through the skin.

DEAD SEA SALT

These contain a rich mixture of over 21 essential nutrients with ten times more life-enhancing natural minerals than table salt. Valuable natural minerals include magnesium, calcium, potassium, sulphur, bromide, iodine, sodium and zinc. Magnesium helps protect and repair the skin; calcium helps renew skin cells; potassium helps balance moisture levels. These essential minerals are absorbed through your skin when you add them to the bath. Dead Sea salt aids in the treatment of common dry, itchy skin problems, such as eczema and psoriasis, and it cleanses, softens and heals blemished skin conditions. Known to reduce pain and inflammation from muscular strain, arthritis and rheumatism when used regularly, it is detoxifying for the entire system while simultaneously replenishing the body with essential minerals.

EPSOM SALT

A pure mineral compound of magnesium sulfate crystals – a natural compound found in water containing high levels of magnesium and sulphate. Many people are magnesium deficient, so it is beneficial to add Epsom salt to a bath regularly, as magnesium is absorbed naturally through the skin. The high levels of magnesium can also help release tension in the muscles, which can be the cause of back pain or stiffness. Epsom salt provides a key function in recovery from sports injuries, swollen joints, cramps or sprains. Magnesium crystals also help maintain normal heart rhythms and can reduce high blood pressure. The salt has a relaxing effect on the whole body, aiding relaxation and soothing general aches and pains – as well as reducing pain and inflammation due to arthritis or rheumatism.

HIMALAYAN
SALT

Known to be one of the purest forms of salt available. It comes in different colours including white, orange and pink and contains more than 80 different minerals, mainly magnesium, iron, potassium and calcium, plus many trace elements. It is sourced from the foothills of the Himalayas, originally the site of ancient salt beds. Himalayan salt has anti-inflammatory properties that calm and soothe the skin while the antimicrobial properties help treat acne, rashes and other skin-related diseases. Using Himalayan salt in the bath regularly aids eczema and psoriasis by reducing skin irritation, redness and swelling. Having antimicrobial and antifungal properties, it is good for haircare – it can help eliminate dandruff and other scalp-related problems. As an exfoliant, it removes dead skin cells while the minerals protect, nourish and rejuvenate the skin. **Note:** Use in moderation due to environmental issues.

SEA
SALT

Distinct from table salt in taste, texture and processing, sea salt is a general term for salt produced by evaporation of ocean water or water from saltwater lakes and is less processed than table salt, retaining many trace minerals – it is commonly available as a kitchen salt in either fine grains or coarse crystals. Natural sea salt is loaded with sodium, which aids hydration of the skin and is essential for the body to maintain a proper fluid balance, transmit nerve impulses and to assist muscle contraction and relaxation. Sea salt also helps cleanse the pores of the skin, while balancing oil production and retaining moisture from within. Its antibacterial properties discourage the growth of bacteria responsible for breakouts and acne. Sea salt exfoliates the skin naturally, while its minerals nourish the skin, making it a good ingredient for body masks and scrubs.

OTHER NATURAL INGREDIENTS

ACTIVATED
CHARCOAL

Activated charcoal is a very effective adsorbent, drawing out impurities from deep within the skin, leaving it ultra clean. The antibacterial properties help reduce acne and improve the overall complexion by lifting bacteria, dirt and oils from the pores. Other visible benefits are that it shrinks the pores and tightens the skin. Moreover, due to its incredible exfoliating properties, it helps shed dead skin cells, making even the appearance of dark spots less visible. Charcoal is an inert material, so it doesn't cause allergic reactions or irritate sensitive skin. Best used in face masks and cleansers to reduce acne and to create a clearer complexion – but it is also good for whitening the teeth! **Note:** Do not use daily as it can absorb the natural oils and moisture in your skin.

BEESWAX

Conditions and calms the skin by creating a hydrating, long-lasting protective barrier against environmental pollutants. It can be used to exfoliate, repair damage and promote cellular regeneration. Antibacterial and antifungal, its anti-inflammatory properties also encourage the healing of wounds. The carotene present in beeswax is a valuable source of vitamin A, which delays collagen degradation and aids faster regeneration of the skin after damage. By acting as a protective, breathable layer on the outer dermis, beeswax helps to lock in moisture. Vegan alternatives include coconut or candelilla wax.

CASTILE
SOAP

A nontoxic, olive oil-based hard or liquid soap named after the Castile region in Spain where it was historically first produced using the local olive and laurel oils. It removes grease effectively and is an ideal ingredient for making all kinds of hair, skin and household cleaning products.

COCONUT
MILK

With many of the nutritional benefits of coconut oil, but less greasy and dense, the milk is suitable for all skin types. It contains lauric acid, decanoic acid, caprylic acid and caproic acid, which are what help to make it such an effective multipurpose product. The milk is very gentle and soothing with good antimicrobial, antiviral and anti-inflammatory properties, which makes it ideal in rinse-off cleansers and masks as well as leave-on moisturizers. It is an all-natural way to deal with sunburn or to reduce any temporary redness, and can help in the treatment of dry and irritated skin conditions like eczema and psoriasis.

COFFEE GRANULES

Naturally full of antioxidants, these have an excellent exfoliating action when applied to the skin in scrubs or masks. The caffeine and chlorogenic acids can help reduce inflammation due to skin problems such as eczema, acne and psoriasis. Additionally, coffee grounds may help fight skin infection given the antimicrobial properties in the beans and there is some indication that coffee applied locally may help reduce the appearance of cellulite.

GLYCERINE

An outstanding moisturizer and skin cleanser that also provides softening and lubricating benefits, vegetable glycerine is a simple, all-natural product that adds moisturizing, cleansing and softening properties to a recipe and is easily soluble in water, but does not mix readily with vegetable oils. For cosmetic use, glycerine also has anti-ageing benefits and can help even out skin tone and texture. As a first aid agent, it can soothe inflammation and facilitate the healing of minor injuries, such as scratches, cuts and infections and promote wound healing. **Note:** Vegetable glycerine is made from natural fats found in botanical or plant-based oils, while another common form is animal-based; always ensure you are using the plant-based type.

HONEY

One of nature's most revered skin remedies due to its natural moisturizing properties, honey is suitable for all skin types, including blemished skin, as it is highly effective in helping to get rid of blackheads by thoroughly cleansing the pores without disrupting the skin's pH balance. It has good antiseptic and antibacterial properties, and since it can easily penetrate the skin, it works to remove any impurities from deep within the pores. The natural antioxidants present in honey improve the skin's elasticity, help delay the signs of ageing and reduce the appearance of wrinkles and fine lines on the face. It imparts a smoother, tighter and healthy glow to the complexion. Honey can help soothe conditions such as eczema and psoriasis, plus it has good exfoliating properties. **Note:** Honey may not be the best choice for you if you are strictly vegan. Those who have pollen allergies should stay away from it too.

JOJOBA BEADS

Made from the liquid wax derived from the jojoba shrub, then processed into a solid wax, or jojoba ester, which is made into spherical beads, jojoba beads are 100 per cent biodegradable and make a great ingredient for exfoliation products, leaving the skin healthy, soft and glowing. They are an eco-friendly alternative to the synthetically produced plastic microbeads commonly found in all sorts of cosmetic products today, which are not biodegradable and are polluting seas, rivers and oceans, plus poisoning and endangering marine life.

OATMEAL AND OAT MILK

Both have outstanding benefits for the skin, particularly when it comes to dry, itchy skin and flare-ups of conditions such as eczema, dermatitis and psoriasis. Oats contain proteins, vitamin E, betaglucan and carbohydrates, plus they have excellent emollient and antioxidant qualities. All these work together to reduce inflammation and irritation when added to a bath, for example, while locking in moisture, making the skin feel supple, soft and soothed. Colloidal oatmeal can be bought ready-made or made at home by grinding oats into a finely milled consistency in a pestle and mortar or food processor or blender. Like oatmeal, oat milk is also very mild on the skin and has been used for centuries to treat dry, itchy skin conditions and rashes, but it is only recently that researchers have discovered it is a phenolic alkaloid called avenanthramide in the oats that is responsible for soothing the skin so effectively.

ROSEHIP POWDER

Extracted from the seeds of wild rose plants and known for its high concentration of vitamin C, which is one of the most potent antioxidants, rosehip powder also contains high levels of vitamins E, A and D together with other nutrients, which vitally improve skin health. Like rosehip oil, the powder is valuable for soothing redness or skin irritations, having excellent anti-inflammatory properties. It contains fatty acids, such as linoleic acid, alpha-linoleic acid and oleic acid, which lock moisture into the skin. The essential fatty acids and antioxidants give it a unique ability to combat UV damage by the sun, treating pigmentation and improving the texture of the skin, while also preventing scarring and encouraging skin regeneration.

RUBBING ALCOHOL

A convenient solvent for making concentrated aromatic products, because essentials oils dissolve readily in alcohol. In most cases, a pure 100-proof vodka can be substituted for rubbing alcohol – but since it is very dehydrating for the skin, it should not applied locally to the body.

SEA MOSS

Sea moss creates a protective layer on the skin and has good moisturizing and nutritional properties thanks to its high concentration of vitamin A, zinc and sulphur. Its antimicrobial and anti-inflammatory properties can help combat acne and blemished skin, and balance oil production. When applied as a mask, it has a soothing quality that can help treat eczema, dermatitis and psoriasis. The vitamin K present helps promote the skin's elasticity and collagen production – this plumps up the skin and smooths wrinkles.

SEAWEED EXTRACT

Containing over 70 vitamins and minerals, and particularly rich in iodine, seaweed hydrates, conditions and helps reduce visible signs of oxidative stress in the skin; the amino acids plump up the skin, improving its elasticity and smoothing out fine lines. Seaweed also contains niacin, which is good for hyperpigmentation, and thanks to its ability to promote collagen production, it is excellent for anti-ageing skincare. Because the cellular structure of seaweed is similar to skin cells, it can help maintain the skin's natural pH balance. It has been shown to help a range of conditions associated with inflammation, like acne, rosacea and eczema. The collagen within seaweed is also a source of hyaluronic acid, which acts as a lubrication agent for hair and skin.

SOAPWORT

A natural botanical material that is both a gentle and powerful cleaning agent. It doesn't take a very strong concentration to function as an effective shampoo or facial cleanser, particularly suitable for delicate complexions. It can be used for treating dry, itchy and sensitive skin.

SUGAR

Brown sugar has an effective skin regenerative action and is a lovely ingredient for scrubs, having a delightful grainy feel. It also helps rehydrate the skin while the glycolic acid present helps diminish scars and can control melanin formation, thus helping to prevent age spots. Brown sugar naturally exfoliates the skin and removes dead cells, but since it is only mildly abrasive, it makes it a good choice for sensitive skin. It hydrates the skin, promoting circulation, and is cleansing, which can be helpful for the treatment of acne.

VINEGAR

Apple cider vinegar has powerful antimicrobial properties that can help ease skin infections and soothe irritation. As a mild acid, it can also help restore the natural pH balance of the skin and keep the skin moisturized – it may even help to lighten hyperpigmentation. It makes a great hair rinse too, balancing the hair and scalp pH plus closing the hair cuticles, which makes hair shinier and easier to detangle.

MINERALS

Some of the principal qualities of the most common minerals found in natural materials such as salts and clays – and also in seaweed and botanical oils – are as follows.

BORON

Builds muscle mass, increases brain activity, strengthens bones and helps wounds heal.

CALCIUM

Helps to keep the bones strong to prevent osteoporosis and is essential for the healthy functioning of many organs, such as the heart. Calcium requires the presence of phosphorus, magnesium and vitamins D and K for adequate absorption. A calcium deficiency may contribute to conditions such as osteoporosis, hypertension and high cholesterol.

CHLORIDE

Needed for maintaining our metabolism – the process of turning food into energy. Chloride also works alongside sodium, potassium and carbon dioxide to maintain the acid–base balance in the body and to keep a proper balance of fluids.

IODINE

Vital for skin repair. Apart from regulating the skin's moisture levels, iodine also aids healing of scars, cuts and minor abrasions. It helps in the regeneration of the lower layers of the skin by triggering important cellular functions resulting in a regular complete rejuvenation of skin, hair and nails.

IRON

Builds up the quality of the blood, prevents stress and fatigue and improves skin tone. It also builds resistance to disease and aids in muscle function. Iron is lost during menstruation, so it is important to replace depleted iron following a period.

MAGNESIUM

Helps build bones, enables proper nerve and muscle function, supports the metabolism and is also necessary for proper enzymatic production. It eases many common complaints, such as headaches, chronic pain, asthma and sleep disorders. Magnesium also helps maintain normal heart rhythms, assists in reducing high blood pressure and has been linked to a reduced incidence of conditions such as heart disease, hypertension and diabetes.

PHOSPHORUS — The second most abundant mineral in our body after calcium, it helps build strong teeth and bones, filters out waste via the kidneys and helps our body store and use energy. Phosphorus plays an active role in tissue and cell growth and repair so it is vital for regeneration of the skin.

POTASSIUM — Active in muscle-nerve communications and in moving nutrients into cells while moving wastes out of the cells. This element assists in the normalization of heart rhythms, reduces high blood pressure, helps to eliminate body toxins and promotes healthy skin.

SILICA — Silica has been shown to contribute to enzyme activities that are necessary for normal collagen formation. Collagen is found in our skin, ligaments and tendons and is essential for maintaining youthful-looking skin. Silica is also vital for maintaining the health of connective tissues, due to its interaction with the formation of glycosaminoglycans. One well-known glycosaminoglycan is hyaluronic acid, which has been shown to promote skin cell proliferation and increase the presence of retinoic acid, improving the skin's appearance. This is now a key ingredient in many skincare products aimed at slowing down the signs of ageing and for maintaining a smooth, wrinkle-free complexion.

SODIUM — Essential for our body to maintain a proper fluid balance, transmit nerve impulses and assist in muscle contraction and relaxation. Natural salts assist with the alleviation of arthritic symptoms, stimulate the body's lymphatic system and also help to maintain the body's fluid balance.

SULPHUR — One of the most plentiful minerals, which is found primarily near hot springs and volcanic craters, sulphur works with vitamins B1 (thiamine), B5 (pantothenic acid) and H (biotin) to promote metabolism and communication between nerve cells. It is most concentrated in keratin, found in strong hair and nails. It is known as 'nature's beauty mineral' because it is essential for the manufacture of collagen, which keeps skin elastic and young-looking. Sulphur also helps soothe itchy skin and conditions such as eczema, psoriasis, dermatitis, dandruff, eczema and warts. In addition, it has been shown to lower cholesterol and blood pressure and ease arthritic pain.

SAFETY GUIDELINES + MEASUREMENTS

Although essential oils, vegetable oils, waxes, botanical herbs, salts and clay are all 100 per cent natural materials, the term 'natural' does not always equate to 'safe'. A few plants are extremely poisonous, such as deadly nightshade (*Atropa belladonna*) and there are also several herbs and oils that should only be used with caution. Valerian oil (*Valeriana officinalis*), for example, should not be used for prolonged periods of time, especially by those suffering from depression. Some essential oils are not recommended for therapeutic use at all due to their high toxicity levels, such as mugwort oil (*Artemisia vulgaris*). Others can cause skin irritation or sensitization in some individuals. Phototoxicity can be an issue, especially in essential oils produced by expression from the peel of certain members of the citrus family, such as grapefruit oil — this can cause skin pigmentation if applied in concentration to areas of the skin which is then exposed to direct sunlight.

The measurements of some materials, such as salts and clays, are not as critical when you are making recipes as there are few contraindications. Vegetable oils and butters are generally safe to apply externally, although those with nut allergies should avoid the use of some products such as coconut, apricot or peach kernel oils. Herbs need to be handled with care, even when making water or oil infusions for external application. Essential oils are extremely concentrated substances, so using the correct measurements is vital. Only a very few oils, such as lavender oil, can be applied directly to the skin in a neat form. Always do a patch test when using an essential oil for the first time. Buy materials from a reputable supplier to ensure they are effective and safe, since they are commonly adulterated with synthetic substitutes.

When using essential oils, it is therefore very important always to take the following simple precautions:

○ Do not take essential oils internally – they are extremely concentrated and can be harmful!

○ In general, essential oils should not be applied undiluted to the skin, although there are a few exceptions to the rule (such as lavender).

○ Do not use essential oils on newborn babies and note that some oils are contraindicated for infants (children under six years of age). Always use the essential oils at half the recommended dilution for children under 12.

○ Some oils should be avoided during pregnancy, others during the first four months only. Always use at half dilution during pregnancy.

○ Some oils should be avoided when in combination with drinking alcohol or using homeopathic remedies, and in cases of high blood pressure, epilepsy or allergies.

○ Do not use essential oils at home to treat serious or longstanding medical or psychological problems — if in doubt, consult a doctor or qualified therapist.

○ Store essential oils in dark bottles, away from light and heat, and well out of the reach of children.

○ Avoid contact with the eyes and delicate areas of the skin. Rinse immediately with plenty of cold water in cases of irritation.

GENERAL CONVERSIONS

1 teaspoon	=	5 grams/5 ml
1 tablespoon	=	15 grams/15 ml
4 teaspoons	=	20 grams/20 ml
1½ tablespoons	=	22.5 grams/22.5 ml
5 teaspoons	=	25 grams/25 ml

ESSENTIAL OIL MEASUREMENTS

There are approximately 20 drops in 1 ml of essential oil.

Millilitres / Ounces		Drops
3.75 ml (⅛ fl oz)	=	75 drops
7.5 ml (¼ fl oz)	=	150 drops
15 ml (½ fl oz)	=	300 drops
30 ml (1 fl oz)	=	600 drops

BLENDING CHART

Recommended drops essential oil for quantities of carrier, or base, oil.

Carrier Oil Quantities	10ml	15ml	25ml	50ml	100ml
Essential Oils % in Drops					
Facial oil (1–1.5%)	1–3	4–5	6–9	12–17	20–28
Body or massage oil (2.5–3%)	5–7	6–8	12–15	25–30	50–60
Perfume blend oil (5%+)	12+	14+	25+	50+	100+
Pregnancy oil (1%)	2	4	6	12	24

AGE GUIDELINES

The following proportions are recommended by age for a body or massage oil using a carrier oil with essential oils.

Age	Amount of carrier oil	Drops of essential oils
65 years +	25 ml	5–8 drops
12–65 years	25 ml	12–15 drops
6–12 years	25 ml	7–10 drops
4–6 years	25 ml	5–7 drops
1–4 years	25 ml	2–3 drops
under 1 year	25 ml	1 drop
0–6 months	25ml	none

Note: Do not use essentials oils on babies under six months. Apricot kernel or peach kernel oil is recommended for sensitive skin.

FURTHER RESOURCES

AQUA OLEUM LTD

Unit 9, Griffin Mill Industrial Estate
London Road, Thrupp, Stroud,
Gloucestershire, GL5 2AZ
United Kingdom

Supplier of premium quality essential oils, vegetable oils and a wide range of other aromatherapy products, including clays and salts. Aqua Oleum Ltd has a heritage spanning over three generations, based on expert family knowledge of essential oils. It was founded by Kerttu Ajanko and is today owned by her daughter Julia Lawless and her granddaughter Natasha. For over 50 years, it has built its market reputation based on outstanding product expertise and high ethical standards, together with a real commitment to providing premium quality oils at a fair price. All Aqua Oleum essential oils have any contraindication clearly stated on the label alongside instructions for use

Website: aqua-oleum.co.uk
General enquiries: info@aqua-oleum.co.uk
Tel: (+44) 01453 885 908

20A BOTANICAL WORKSHOPS

Hands-on workshops in aromatherapy blending, bespoke products and botanically based recipes. Founded by Abi Titterington Lough, 20A strives to educate and inspire individuals through the medium of aromatherapy and to foster a sense of curiosity, creativity and involvement in our own wellbeing. Through interactive in-person and online workshops, courses and consultations, 20A experiences explore the full spectrum of a plant's potential to support you holistically.

Website: 20a.co
General enquiries: abi@20a.co

JEKKA'S HERB FARM

Rose Cottage, Shellards Lane, Alveston,
Bristol, BS35 3SY United Kingdom

Suppliers of herbs, seeds and ongoing education advice on using and growing a wide range of herbs. Founded by Jekka McVicar, Jekka's Herb Farm in Somerset has been described as 'a living book of herbs' and offers a variety of educational and inspiring aromatic experiences for the amateur, enthusiast and professional. Open days, workshops and talks at Jekka's provide a way to learn about growing sustainable culinary and medicinal herbs, as well as how to use them.

Website: jekkas.com
Email: sales@jekkas.com
Tel: (+44) 01454 418 878

FURTHER READING

Several of the books listed here have been published in various editions and translated into different languages. Signed copies of many of Julia's books can be bought from the Aqua Oleum website. Most of her books are available from good bookstores while some are also available as e-books, including her all-time bestselling aromatherapy classic: *The Encyclopedia of Essential Oils*.

Aloe Vera: Natural Wonder Cure, Julia Lawless & Judith Allan (Thorsons, 2000).

Aromatherapy and the Mind, Julia Lawless (Thorsons, 1995).

The Blending Notebook: An Introduction to the Art of Formulating Your Own Aromatic Creations, Julia Lawless (London stationers Mark + Fold). Available from Aqua Oleum.

The Complete Aromatherapy & Essential Oils Sourcebook, Julia Lawless (Harper Collins, 2017).

The Complete Essential Oil Sourcebook, Julia Lawless (Harper Collins, 2016).

The Complete Illustrated Guide to Aromatherapy, Julia Lawless (Thorsons, 1998).

The Encyclopedia of Essential Oils, Julia Lawless (Harper Collins, 1992). New revised and extended edition published in 2014.

The Essential Aromatherapy Garden, Julia Lawless (Thorsons, 2019).

Essential Oils: An Illustrated Guide, Julia Lawless (Thorsons, 2002).

The Fragrant Garden: Growing and Using Scented Plants, Julia Lawless (Kyle Cathie, 2005).

Heaven Scent: Aromatic Christmas Crafts, Recipes and Decorations, Julia Lawless (Element, 1998).

Home Aromatherapy, Julia Lawless (Kyle Cathie, 1995).

The Home Use of Essential Oils (booklet), Julia Lawless, available from Aqua Oleum Ltd.

The Illustrated Encyclopedia of Essential Oils, Julia Lawless (Element, 1995).

Lavender Oil: Nature's Soothing Herb, Julia Lawless (Thorsons, 2001).

Rose Oil: Nature's Most Precious Perfume & Traditional Remedy, Julia Lawless (Thorsons, 2014).

Rosemary Oil: Nature's Most Revitalizing Remedy, Julia Lawless (Thorsons, 2014).

Tea Tree Oil: One of Nature's Most Remarkable Gifts, Julia Lawless (Thorsons, 2001).

INDEX

AUTHOR ACKNOWLEDGEMENTS

I would like to thank my mother Kerttu for inspiring my enduring love for nature and especially for my interest in herbs and essential oils; my daughter Natasha for her help with imagery and her outstanding photographic skills; my granddaughter Anouk for her endless enthusiasm for making, blending and creating; Abi Titterington Lough for her beauty and skincare expertise and invaluable collaboration on recipe formulation; all my colleagues at Aqua Oleum for their ongoing commitment and support; Marianne Sheehan for her helpful comments on the draft text; Lisa Dyer my commissioning editor for being such a pleasure to work with; and Georgie Hewitt for her excellent book design and layout.

PICTURE CREDITS

The publishers would like to thank the following sources for their kind permission to reproduce the pictures in this book.

Courtesy of Aqua Oleum: 26, 53, 152.
Getty Images: Ashlynne Lobdell / EyeEm 36; Cavan Images 136; Chris Griffiths 90; Gwenvidig 142; honey_ and_milk 68; Jupiterimages 39; Kazmulka 30; Madeleine_Steinbach 128; Olgaorly 29; Park Lane Pictures 55; Pra Phasr Xaw Sakhr / EyeEm 127. **Pexels:** Alesia Kozik 65, 86; Cottonbro 35, 82; Karolina Grabowska 88, 105, 107; Monstera 27, 32, 51; Nana Lapushkina 52; Pavel Danilyuk 43, 85; RF studio 95; Rodnae Productions 14, 96; Tara Winstead 42, 50, 132; Yan Krukov 12, 123. **Shutterstock:** Anna Gawlik 109; gorillaimages 112; images72 120; Ira Sokolovskaya 130; Ivan_Shenets 80; JPC-PROD 28; Konstantinos Livadas 84; Maridav 61; New Africa 41; nito 62; Number1411 102; Pixel-Shot 121; Rido 57; Shamils 135; Shishkin.dv 63; Valeriya Zankovych 94. **Unsplash:** Adrien Olichon 15, 137; Alaksiej Carankievic 108; Andrii Leonov 160; Annie Spratt 4, 118; Atle Mo 11; Content Pixie 111; crystalweed 78; Erwan Hesry 138; Fulvio Ciccolo 87; Georgie de Lotz 3; Huha Inc 72; Jernej Graj 75; Joshua Freake 24; Kadarius Seegars 58; Lindsay Moe 79; Logan Fisher 16; Miguel Bruna 146; Monika Kozub 124; Nathan Dumlao 34; Paje Victoria 25; Rasa Kasparaviciene 119; Robert Gomez 21; Rodolfo Sanches Carvalho 44; ruralexplorer 6; Sara Scarpa 129; Sarah Janes 40; Taisiia Stupak 49, 125; Toa Heftiba 93; Tron Le 131; Volant 104.